PROSTATE CANCER
DECODED

Newer Life-Saving
Prostate Cancer Treatments

Robert L. Bard, MD

Morgan James Publishing • New York

PROSTATE CANCER DECODED

Disclaimer
The information in this book is for educational purposes only and is not a substitute for professional medical care.
—Dr. Robert Bard and The Biofoundation for Angiogenesis R&D

Library of Congress Number: 2007935482
Paperback ISBN: 978-1-60037-346-6

Printed in the United States of America

Books Co-Authored by Dr. Bard
ULTRASONOGRAPHY OF THE ABDOMEN
ULTRASONOGRAPHY OF THE PELVIS
ULTRASONOGRAPHY OF THE EYE
DECONSTRUCTING PROSTATE CANCER
PROSTATE CANCER DEMYSTIFIED

Published by:

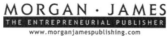

www.morganjamespublishing.com

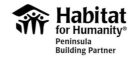
Habitat for Humanity®
Peninsula
Building Partner

Morgan James Publishing, LLC
1225 Franklin Ave. Ste 325
Garden City, NY 11530-1693
Toll Free 800-485-4943
www.MorganJamesPublishing.com

Cover and Interior Design by:
Michelle Radomski
One to One Creative Services
www.creativeones.net

To my patients, whose courage showed me possibility
To my wife, Loreto, whose vision generated reality

You see things: and you say, "Why?"
But I dream things that never were: and say, "Why not?"
—George Bernard Shaw

ACKNOWLEDGMENTS

I thank Loreto Bard, Executive Director of the Biofoundation for Angiogenesis Research and Development, for her assistance in coordinating international multidisciplinary medical exchanges that advanced the concepts developed in this book. I wish to thank members of: the Prostate Cancer Research Institute; Drs. Duke Bahn, Stanley Brosman, Arthur Lurvey, Mark Scholz and Charles Myers; members of the Catholic University Hospital in Rome, Italy, Drs. Giuseppe Brisinda, Federica Cadeddu and Giorgio Maria: members of the Mayo Clinic Foundation, Drs. Thayne Larson, Benjamin Larson and Lance Mynderse: member of the Academic Hospital of Bicetre, Dr.Francoise Giuliano: members of The Prostatitis Foundation, Drs. Susan Keay and John Warren: members of the NY Roentgen Society, Drs. Richard Stock, Lincoln Pao, Michael Zelefsky, Alan Pollack, Shalom Kalnicki: members of the Societe Francaise de Radiologie, Drs. Guy Frija, Olivier Helenon, JF Moreau and JM Correas; members of the Paul Morel Hospital, Vesoul, France, Drs. JL Sauvain, R Palasac and P. Palasac; members of the Instituto Radiologia, Policlinico Umberto I, Rome, Drs. Plinio Rossi, Roberto Passariello and Vito Cantisani: members of the Groupe Hospitalier Necker-Enfants Malades, Paris, France, Drs. Bertrand Dufour, N. Thiounn, JM Correas and Y. Chretien; members of the Imperial College of Medicine, London, Dr. David Cosgrove and Sir Richard Sykes; members of the American Urological Association, Drs. Carl Olsson, William DeWolf, Edward Messing, Louis Denis, Eric Rovner, Ernest Sosa, Alexis Te, Michael Manyak, Michael Marberger, Joseph Smith, Jr, Harris Nagler, J. Fracchia, Peter Scardino, M. Droller, P. Schlegel, S. Kaplan, H. Lepor, M. Grasso, N. Romas, A. Melman, I. Grunberger, R. Macchia, M. Choudhury and Patrick Walsh; members of the New York Cancer Society, Drs. Marvin Rotman and Howard Hochster. Dr. Jelle Barentsz, president of the International Cancer Imaging Society, for developing lymph node detection technology and disseminating awareness throughout the medical profession. Special thanks to Drs. Catherine Roy, Francois Cornud, Olivier Helenon, Mitchell Gaynor, Peter Scardino, Ralph Moss and Majid Ali whose books have provided new hope for cancer victims and further advanced medical knowledge.

AUTHOR'S BACKGROUND

Diplomat American Board of Radiology
Member American College of Radiology
Clinical Assistant Professor of Radiology New York Medical College
Director, Bio-foundation for Angiogenesis Research and Development
Advisory Board, International Musculoskeletal Ultrasound Society
High Intensity Focused Ultrasound Certification—Prostate Cancer Imaging
Member, International Cancer Imaging Society

PROLOGUE

Summer, 1949. Polio ward. Helen Hayes Hospital. New York State.

First the breathing got harder. Then the fingers turned blue. I was paralyzed from the waist down with acute poliomyelitis and I now feared my diaphragms were failing. The doctors at the rehabilitation center specializing in this nationwide epidemic had already warned my parents I would never walk, even though I felt some sensation coming back in my right leg. I could hear the monotonous steady mechanical sounds from the next ward where the "iron lungs" for completely paralyzed children assisted their respiration in hopes they would recover the ability to inhale before they died. The boys I saw sent to the respirator room never came back. I was scared my next ward would be my last stop. I was five years old and worried I would never see my sixth birthday.

Summer, 1949. Dr. Harold Bard's internal medicine practice. New York City.

The phone rang. My father's face turned white. He told the receptionist to cancel the afternoon patients. He called my mother and told her it was such a beautiful day that they would take a drive to the country to see their son recovering from paralytic polio. My father, a bronze star medal winner as a physician during World War II, came in to examine me. He heard me cough, saw my dusky color, listened to my lungs, felt my hot forehead and went over to talk to my doctors. There was arguing. My father told the physician in charge I had acute pneumonia—they told him I was dying from the paralysis of my diaphragms preventing me from breathing. My father stopped talking to them, came back and whispered to me: "See these little white pills? Take one pill before each meal. Do not tell anyone else you are taking them. I will be back tomorrow." I hid the tablets under my pillow. At meal time I decided to follow my dad's advice and ignore the specialists taking care of me. The next morning my breathing was better. My father had brought back with him the antibiotic penicillin from the Pacific theater of war. It was still not widely available in the United States in 1949 and certainly not well understood. Penicillin saved the GI's lives during the war. My father saved my life by trusting his battle tested experience rather than the advice of the so called experts.

My father studied medicine in Switzerland and was fluent in 7 languages. He was training in surgical subspecialties in New York when World War II broke out. He volunteered to serve his country and went to Pearl Harbor to treat the wounded. He was then sent with the Army Ranger Units to fight with the soldiers in Alaska and, later, in the South Pacific. He fought overseas for 28 months continuously without ever coming home to see his new born son. He fought in the arctic, fought in the jungle, fought in the desert and fought in the mountains. He lived medicine in the raw—he saw all types of injury and disease in the extreme—he improvised to save his soldiers by operating in tents lit by flash lights and kerosene lanterns during counter-attacks. He passed on his passion to develop new medical ideas to his son by example. I might have died prematurely if I had listened to the traditional medical advice of those days.

I volunteered to support my country during the Vietnam conflict. With one year of radiology specialty experience, I was sent to Thailand to support the Tactical Air Command as a Captain in the U.S. Air Force. As the only USAF radiologist within 300 kilometers of Udorn Royal Thai Air Base, I went to far off places to assist in diagnoses that took me to southern Thailand, Laos, Formosa, Guam, Vietnam and Cambodia. The Air Force medical facility at our base took care of the U.S. General Staff and soldiers of our allied forces. This was a "state of the art" military hospital and retained physicians of the highest caliber from all over the US.

I also learned that the practice of medicine was not from a text book. Reality did not coincide with cook book formulations. For example, the treatment of the Cambodian colonel whose chest x-ray revealed multiple live hand-grenades buried in his chest wall could not be found in any medical text book. There were also many different ways to treat diseases within our nation-wide American thinking and even more options employing oriental possibilities. Remember, in China, if the Chinese emperor died, so did his physician. Exposed to varied treatment possibilities, I eagerly tried to integrate eastern medicine concepts with proven western medicine teachings. I soon learned that there were alternative ways to treat many medical problems. I also noted that westerners were physically and emotionally different than oriental peoples. For example, the Thai people would rest by squatting. American's, trying to fit in with local customs, quickly developed knee joint irritations. The make up of their Asian bodies was notably different from our North American physiques. Upon completion of active duty, I returned to the United States as a major and as a man who had seen diseases and treatments not common in traditional medical studies. I was humbled by the inexplicable success of eastern remedies not readily understood by western standards.

FOREWORD

"While MRI is certainly proving valuable, the maturation of 3-D ultrasound will go a long way towards matching MRI'S capabilities," states Dr. B. Benacerraf, Professor of Radiology at Harvard Medical School.

During October 2003, I attended the JOURNEES FRANCAISES DE RADI-OLOGIE in Paris, the major radiology conference in Europe, where I witnessed the potential of 3-Dimensional (3-D) technology for imaging the prostate that also gave computer graphic reconstructions of the capsule (covering) and internal structure, including vasculature (blood vessels) of the prostate gland. Although the equipment was approved for use all over the world, including the United States, there was not one unit being used in North America. As of this writing, I am one of the few physicians using the European designed Voluson ultrahigh resolution multiplanar automatic acquisition 3-D power Doppler ultrasound system in the United States for prostate imaging. The reason is simply that urologists use the sonogram to guide the prostate biopsy and do not take advantage of the advanced technology that offers 3-D imaging like an MRI exam. Internists and family physicians refer patients with prostate problems to urologists. Patients naturally seek urologic assistance as the first step to resolving prostate disorders. Radiologists do not see patients for this type of exam because patients are not referred for radiologic imaging by urologists or family practitioners, in large part because this is a new diagnostic modality.

I am writing this book to inform patients about the cutting edge of medical diagnosis and new therapeutic options using image guided treatments. I have changed my profession from "diagnostic radiologist" who saw only films to "interventional radiologist" who examines a patient and provides therapy based on the current picture of the disease. Treatment may be tailored for each patient based on newer concepts in radiological imaging and on sensitivity to the patient's needs and lifestyle choices.

Life without humor, according to Oscar Wilde, is not worth living. Medicine without compassion may not be worth dispensing. It is too easy today to cure the disease and destroy the patient in the process as we have witnessed with chemotherapies. This book aims at preserving human dignity and controlling cancer at the same time. My purpose for writing this book is to provide practical knowledge of disease, offer hope based on scientific data and realistic empowerment to deal with life's medical adversities.

Not all prostate cancer kills. In fact, many prostate cancers are now treatable without surgery. Minimally invasive treatment for benign diseases can be done in fifteen minutes while minimally invasive definitive cancer treatments may take from one to four hours. But, the message here is that a person need not fear prostate cancer when new and non-invasive modalities are now being utilized to detect malignant tumors quickly, painlessly, and more accurately. The multiplicity of non invasive and minimally invasive therapies with fewer side effects offers men a wider and more palatable array of health choices.

TABLE OF CONTENTS

CHAPTER ONE
New Methods of Detection

---

11 PM. Emergency Department. Metropolitan Hospital. New York City, 1973.
Twenty-six year old female brought in with stab wound to the chest and increasing shortness of breath. Medical team must know if there is blood in the pericardium, the sac that holds the heart. I confer with the heart surgeon, leave the ED and proceed to the obstetrics department. I bring back an ultrasound machine used on a pregnant woman's abdomen for determining fetal growth and place the scanner over the heart of the bleeding patient. With clear images of the extent of the injury, the patient is rushed to the OR. The surgeon, now armed with a precise picture of the site of the hemorrhage, targets his operation. The bleeding around the heart is stopped at 1:00 AM. The patient lives.

This real life story shows even a dedicated medical technology may have multiple potential uses. Eye scanners were used on the breast in 1978 to perceive mammary problems. Breast scanners looked at joints and tendons in 1990. Tendon imaging devices that showed blood vessels and demonstrated actual live blood flow near a joint were adapted to imaging the prostate in the mid 90's. Scanners, showing the face of the fetus using 3-Dimensional (3-D) pictures inside the uterus ten years ago, were soon placed on the shoulder to assess injuries. Technology that improved shoulder imaging with 3-D pictures became available for the prostate five years ago. For a while, medical imaging was mainly limited by the lack of curiosity of the physician and the paucity of semiconductor technology to make more powerful computer chips. Medical breakthroughs are sometimes as simple as thinking outside the box.

The following story of the "Rat and the Cheese" is pertinent to the advancement of science, as it characterizes basic human nature and its effect on scientific discovery. A rat was put in a tunnel with a piece of cheese at the end. The rat ran down the tunnel and ate the cheese. Day after day the rat was able to wend its way down the course to find unerringly the tasty morsel. One day the cheese was removed. The rat went down the tunnel and tried to find the cheese. The next day the rat entered the tunnel and searched without success. The third day the rat went into the tunnel and came out without any cheese. At the end of the fourth day the rat refused to enter the tunnel.

The difference between rats and human beings is—after a while, the rat gives up going down a tunnel with no cheese. The rat re-thought the situation by learning quickly what worked and what did not work. Human beings often continue their behavior patterns in the absence of tangible rewards. For example, if one goes into a room full of people and ask those who are 10 pounds or more overweight to raise their hands, and then ask those who know that exercise and dieting will control their weight to raise their hands—the same hands go up. Do you know how monkeys get caught? You see, these primates are similar to humans in important ways. A banana is put into a jar with a narrow neck. The monkey reaches into the jar and grabs the banana in his closed fist. The width of the clenched hand with the banana is wider than the jar opening. As the hunter comes to catch the monkey, the trapped animal gets worried and agitated, but will not let go of the banana. All it had to do was give up what it was holding on to—simple, but not part of instinctual behavior.

Like the rat analogy, people often behave like other higher order mammals. Men habitually avoid dealing with health issues by denial based on fear. A man's first approach to a medical problem is to wait, hoping it will go away. When the condition worsens, he waits again hoping his health won't deteriorate further. Finally, when he can no longer put up with the alteration of his lifestyle or the intolerance of his physical state, he decides to get help. FEAR stops men from being proactive in their health. Women complain bitterly about the pain of mammograms, yet few miss their yearly appointments. In New York City the current wait for this despised test is up to 4 months.

What's behind the fear of seeing the doctor? Most patients fall into five categories:
1. The stoic: who sees sickness as unmanly—a sign of weakness
2. The worrier: who knows too much about possible medical side effects
3. The ostrich: who is in denial
4. The victim: who gets attention from others
5. The perfect patient: who attends to potential problems early

Fear is a physiologic byproduct of incipient thwarted intention of our natural need for survival. Seeing a doctor activates our concerns over pain, interruption of daily routine, recovery and, possibly, death. White collar hypertension is a real phenomenon.

Our blood pressure often rises in the doctor's office with the stress of a possible serious medical condition. A few deep breaths may bring the numbers back to normal. The same phenomenon is true with glaucoma, high pressure in the eye. Most patients hold their breath as the metal probe advances towards the eye ball. This falsely elevates the internal ocular reading. Relaxing and breathing usually lowers the number to a safe level. Other causes of fear in the doctor's office are bad childhood experiences, claustrophobia, fear of needles, fainting at the sight of blood, low pain threshold, cold examination rooms, exposing parts of the body, etc.

No matter what kind of patient you are and no matter what your fear of the unknown, don't wait till it is too late. Tell the physician and his staff about your anxiety and request specific arrangements. While no one objects to a prostate sonogram, most men wince at the thought of being inside the claustrophobic MRI tube for half an hour. For these concerns, we may modify the procedure to keep the head outside the tube or inject anti-anxiety medicine to reduce the stress of the procedure.

For example, a colleague in good health developed heartburn and treated it with antacids for two weeks. When it got worse and the acid rose up in his throat irritating the voice box producing hoarseness, he called the gastroenterologist. The GI doctor told him to fast after midnight and see him at 8 AM the next morning for an endoscopy—a scope inserted through the mouth that looks at the esophagus and stomach. He had a light dinner and started the fast earlier at 10 PM. After the anesthesia wore off from the procedure, he was told the test couldn't be performed because the stomach had not emptied and the retained food contents blocked the view of the endoscope. He knew in a flash that common causes for an obstruction preventing emptying of the stomach was either a severe duodenal ulcer or cancer of the outlet end of the stomach. Since he had no real pain, he was sure he had a malignancy. He consulted me and we arrived at the understanding that worst possible outcome, cancer, might still be in an early stage. The test was repeated after a 12 hour fast and a small benign ulcer of the stomach wall was discovered which resolved in a month under routine treatment. The moral is: it is better to deal with your worst nightmare promptly than to procrastinate and lose the opportunity for curative treatment. The ancient philosopher, Seneca, said *"pars sanitatis velle sanari fuit"* or "the wish to be cured is part of the cure"

Physicians are human, too. While we try to do the best for our patients, doctors are slow to give up customary ideas and even slower to accept new concepts. Medical practitioners rightfully demand proof that a change from a tried and true routine will make sense before adopting a new method. My former partner and late colleague, Dr. Selig Strax, Professor of Surgery at Mount Sinai Medical Center in New York also commented on the tendency of the medical profession's avoidance of change. He had introduced the first "lumpectomy" operation for breast conservation at Mount Sinai half a century ago. It took a quarter century for this proven method to be uniformly adopted throughout the national medical community. The original radical mastectomy surgical operation, removing the entire breast, chest wall muscles, and occasionally part of the rib cage, was based on the 100 year old idea that cancer spread like a crab to local organs. After the discovery that small cancers could spread to the lymph nodes (glands) and to every other organ through the blood stream, did the radical mastectomy cease? No. For the next thirty years this mutilating procedure was the gold standard of breast cancer therapy in spite of growing proof that it had outlived its purpose. Women of the last quarter century didn't have this information easily available to them. Today's man is armed with the internet, the news media and varied support groups. Men need not acquiesce to a specified treatment or dictated therapy. The information revolution allows them to choose the best available medical options for their particular condition and level of comfort with the stated potential risks. Einstein once said: "imagination is more important than knowledge"

If I propose the "prostate lumpectomy," how long will it take for the scientific community to even consider the possibility? This book offers options to routine medical care in the United States, and proposes simple, straightforward and logical alternatives to current "gold standard" accepted treatments. Many of these diagnostic modalities and therapeutic procedures are common practice in Europe and other countries with advanced socialized medicine around the civilized world.

There are two important phrases in classic scientific methodology: clinical trial and anecdotal observation. Clinical trial is evidence accumulated based on an assumption of a possible mechanism of therapy to be investigated. Anecdotal observation means that a treatment worked once or twice, and the mechanism may not be readily understood at that time. The bard of modern times says, "To succeed, or not to succeed; that is the question." **It is more useful to have a treatment that works and is not understood than to have a therapy that makes sense but ultimately fails.** A beef steak placed over a black eye helps, however, the cold and pressure of an ice pack would do better to reduce the pain and swelling. Likewise, dabbing tincture of iodine over a cut will sterilize the wound but produce more tissue damage due to its high local toxicity.

David Hess in the Rutgers *University Press* publication, (1999) "Evaluating Alternative Cancer Therapies" quotes the following from medical scholar Robert Houson:

The FDA requires a convincing mechanism to obtain approval for clinical trials, and I think this is a completely unnecessary requirement. If there are indications of benefit in humans or animals, that should bypass the whole issue of mechanism. The point is that the investigators do not have to know the mechanism in order to corroborate the effect that is occurring. In cancer, case studies have a greater degree of validity than in other diseases. In cancer the rate of spontaneous remission is extremely low, so low that it is virtually zero. Therefore, if you have just a few cases, even only two cases, you have something that is significant and most likely meaningful. So, I consider what is being dismissed as anecdotal evidence, to be in cancer, actually an impressive proof of success because you can have much more detail in the case studies than you can in a clinical trial.

In the 1980's, when the state of the art sonogram equipment showed that doctors could see malignant lymph nodes (cancerous glands), I started a protocol with Cabrini Medical Center in New York City under the famed breast surgeon, Dr. Henry Leis. We scanned patients with breast cancer to see if the underarm lymph nodes were involved by tumor. Detection of these cancerous glands meant surgery was not indicated, since abnormal glands showed the cancer had spread too far for a local operation to be useful. The results of our investigation spared selected patients unnecessary surgery. The project showed that the sonogram accurately detected larger cancerous glands, thereby saving some patients from the operating room. We also discovered certain types of highly aggressive breast cancers seemed to shrink the breast instead of producing a lump. In these patients, the mammogram was read as "normal" even though the contracted breast tissue was hard as a rock at the physical examination. This variety of cancer produced scarring and retraction of the tissues as it grew. While the mammogram was useless in the diagnosis, we learned the sonogram visualized them easily. The hospital then began a screening program for high risk patients which led to the discovery of malignancies at very early stages. This has increased the amount of surgery and decreased the spread of cancer resulting in more favorable outcomes. The investigational use of ultrasound technology became a clinical trial after anecdotal cases pointed the way to a specific treatment protocol. The judicious application of the sonographic modality has simultaneously decreased unnecessary surgery and increased curative operations.

My high school chemistry teacher in 1958 was Mr. Marantz. As an eager student, I had looked up some information in a journal and proudly told him I had done some "research" on a topic. He looked at me sternly, saying, "Research is not finding something in a book. Research is being immersed in a project and observing and analyzing what happens during the investigation." He then related his story how he became a school teacher. He was a topnotch industrial research chemist before he entered a teaching career. The New Jersey pharmaceutical plant he worked in was located alongside a river. Three of the walls of the laboratory were steel and concrete. The fourth wall, facing the river, was made of plasterboard and wood. He invented new substances by taking risks and boldly trying unexplored chemical pathways. From time to time there would be a fire or an explosion, and he, the false wall and the experiment would land in the river. After the fourth time and loss of three fingers, he left for the (at the time) safer task of teaching high school students.

I, too, took a risk in forging my path in medicine. After I returned from military service in South East Asia to my radiology residency at the New York Medical College, I requested a leave from the program to attend the renowned Armed Forces Institute of Pathology. The AFIP, as it is commonly referred to, is the national medical teaching center specializing in correlating radiologic findings with unusual pathologic specimens. The chief of my residency allowed me three months unpaid leave to study in Washington, D.C. My experience of reviewing selected cases from the US Armed Forces referred in from the military's world wide theaters of operation gave me a particular edge in interpreting x-rays. I remember vividly in 1973 the director of the radiology training program showed a difficult case of gonococcus urethritis (venereal disease of the male urethra) at the afternoon teaching conference, and I was the only resident who made the diagnosis because of my specific experiences in the military and my correlational training at the AFIP. In disbelief, the director commented aloud that I must have seen the films beforehand in the urology clinic of the hospital. As my third year was finishing, it was the custom of the department head to sit with the residents and guide them to their future. The chief completely dismissed my enthusiasm for the new field of diagnostic ultrasound as "impractical." I took a risk, just like my chemistry teacher. This time the experiment didn't blow up. I was fortunate that the sonogram has become the primary imaging diagnostic test in use today worldwide. As of this date, many new, previously unthinkable uses are becoming available to the medical community in this rapidly growing diagnostic field that has re-entered the treatment arena by its ability to image guide therapies. Simply said, if a disease or tumor can be imaged by a radiologic procedure, it may be treated under direct visual observation at the same time.

Much of the work I am presenting is both a clinical trial and anecdotal evidence simultaneously studied and accumulated over a twelve year period. During this time the subject has been exhaustively evaluated and ongoingly redesigned as better technologies became available. I saw alternative cancer treatments work in patients. These cancer survivors came in for follow up exams, continuously, every six months to monitor their health. All the men had refused traditional medical therapies and standard surgical regimens. In short order, the mechanism of action of tumor growth revealed itself to me. Also, the possibility to use ultrasound technology for diagnostic evaluation and prognostic information predicting the longevity of the patient became obvious.

The *Rat and the Cheese* analogy helps us understand the mechanism of change in the practice of medicine. Acceptance of new ideas occurs slowly, and its transformation into action as distinct new protocols is frequently glacial. The information presented in this book is not new, is not hidden and is not controversial. The majority of concepts in this book have been in use internationally for over twenty years. The same way that the radical mastectomy was phased out by the breast "lumpectomy," so may the traditional radical prostatectomy pass into history as a treatment that no longer serves the good of most patients. Already the standard treatment to improve urine flow in men with enlarged prostates (the Trans-Urethral Resection of the Prostate or TURP) is becoming less popular amongst younger urologists in training programs.

When Dr. Bertrand Guillonneau introduced the robotic radical prostatectomy procedure in Paris in 1995, he was considered strange to alter the existing established treatment. His student, Dr. Arnon Krongrad, brought this laser surgical technique to the United States in 1999, and was initially outcast by the local medical community. Patients who can drive home a few days after surgery cannot understand why this isn't the new standard of care. Today's patients are not passive. Educated patients want what *does* work rather than what *should* work.

The drug *finasteride* (Proscar) was developed fifteen years ago as a miracle cure for progressive urinary symptoms of an enlarged prostate. Initial clinical trials showed it was useful and Proscar rapidly received FDA approval. Early studies also suggested that it may reduce the risk of prostate cancer. Anecdotal reports that it was only minimally effective began to appear and increased in number. New data also suggested men were developing serious cancers while on the medication. A critique of a large study recently concluded, surprisingly, that while the drug was somewhat useful in alleviating the symptoms of benign prostatic hypertrophy, and there was an overall 25 percent decrease in prostate cancer prevalence, there was a 68 percent increase in the frequency of high grade killing prostate cancers in the treated group. This report, published in the *2004 Journal of Urology* by Dr. Patrick Walsh of Johns Hopkins Medical Center, underscores the interaction between clinical trials and anecdotal reports. The wonder drug produced fewer non-lethal tumors but stimulated more aggressive killing cancers.

News Tribune, December 10, 2004 reports researchers at California's Stanford University School of Medicine have added to the confusion with new finding that 98 percent of all prostates removed in the last five years at that facility were removed unnecessarily. These operations left about 3 percent of the patients incontinent and at least half with sexual difficulties, including impotency. The news media and increasing numbers of medical articles are shining a needed spotlight on medical practices and scientific beliefs that require transformation. The trend in cancer therapy is turning towards treating the active tumor more aggressively and sparing the non threatening part of the organ.

There is further concern surrounding current acceptable diagnostic and treatment practices, not the least of which is the reliability of the now embattled prostate specific antigen (PSA) blood test. It is time to rethink long-standing and traditional approaches to prostate cancer detection and the efficacy of currently accepted cures.

CHAPTER TWO
Understanding the Facts

A century ago, physicians were taught that cancers started with a few cells that divided, gradually enlarging to become major clusters of actively growing cells called tumors. At a certain size, the tumor would become more aggressive and begin invading adjacent organs and structures spreading out like the tentacles of an octopus. The concept of blood borne distant metastasizing (spreading) of a local tumor appeared years later. This theory did not explain the fact that some breast and prostate cancers would appear and remain stable over periods of up to thirty-five years without growing or metastasizing. Fifty years ago the colon polyp (small benign growth) was thought to be innocent, until it was learned that certain polyps left untreated eventually turned malignant. There appear to be many shades of gray in our current black or white reality. Modern ideas of cancer generation have continually changed over time. Newer concepts and innovative treatments are presented in the following chapters.

Sometimes physicians accept evidence that does not fully take into consideration the totality of facts at hand, or perhaps, are not cognizant of the overall spectrum of clinical data. I acknowledge generalization is useful and necessarily makes learning easier, but diseases, and patients individually, do not conform to generalities. Let us look at "facts" currently made available to physicians and the public by the media and cancer organizations.

According to American Cancer Society Facts and Figures 2004, 230,000 cases of prostate cancer are diagnosed every year in the United States. Of those, 30,000 men die annually. Findings reported by the Centers for Disease Control and Prevention and the National Cancer Institute in collaboration with the North American Association of Central Cancer Registries show the leading type of cancer causing death among men is lung cancer, however, prostate cancer is the most common form of cancer diagnosed in men in the United States.

Prostate cancer facts:

- One in 6 men will get prostate cancer.
- A man is 33 percent more likely to develop prostate cancer than a woman is to develop breast cancer.
- As baby boomer men reach the target zone for prostate cancer, beginning at age 50, the number of new cases is projected to increase dramatically.
- By 2015, there will be more than 300,000 new prostate cancer cases each year, a 50 percent increase.
- There has been no change in the US cancer death rate between 1950 and 2001.
- In this same time period, there have been decreases in the death rate for other diseases:
  Pneumonia decreased 54%
  Strokes decreased 68%
  Heart disease decreased 58%

The lifetime probability of a man in the US developing cancer is 50 percent.

A breakdown of this data shows the lifetime cancer probability for:

1. Prostate–17%
2. Lung–8%
3. Colon–6%
4. Bladder–3%
5. Lymphoma–2%
6. Melanoma–2%
7. Leukemia–2%
8. Mouth–1%
9. Kidney–1%
10. Stomach–1%

- Men are more likely to develop prostate cancer than all other cancers combined (except lung)
- Prostate cancer is the most common and most rapidly increasing cancer
- Without improvements in diagnosis and treatment:
    1. In 2015 the number of new prostate cancer cases will increase 50%
    2. In 2037 there will be over 400,000 new prostate cancer cases per year

3. In 2020, the number of prostate cancer deaths per year will increase 44%

4. In 2030, 80,000 men will lose their lives to prostate cancer

(Statistical Source: Prostate Cancer Foundation 2004)

News of New York published by the Medical Society of the State of New York reported in the March 2004 issue that:

> While the latest report from the National Cancer Institute (NCI) suggests that death rates for the top cancer killers in men and women are dropping, the lifetime rate of probability of developing cancer remains at 1 in 2 for men and 1 in 3 for women.
>
> The March 23, 2004 issue of the Wall Street Journal in the Health Journal article touched upon this with their piece, "Improve Prostate Cancer Detection, Doctors Change Approach to Testing. What is the change?" To increase the cancer detection rate, a lowering of the threshold for biopsy is recommended. The standard of a level of PSA greater than 4 (normal 0–4 ng/ml) was considered suspicious. Some physicians are saying this is too high to detect cancers and feel a biopsy should be performed when the PSA level is above 2.5. The May 27, 2004 issue of the New York Times reports that even when the PSA is normal, "prostate cells may prove to be cancerous."

A forum on prostate cancer biopsies at the 2004 International Congress of Radiology reported the PSA would often rise following a biopsy, which would lead to another biopsy to determine the reason for the elevated PSA, which would in turn further raise the PSA resulting in another biopsy to rule out cancer based on a rising PSA level. One patient was given a series of six biopsies five different times (totaling 30 punctures) over four years due to rising PSA levels. Cancer was never found. No physician on the panel of experts made the connection that the trauma of the biopsy procedure by itself (not a cancer) may have generated higher PSA levels. (PSA levels are proven to rise due to tumor, trauma, inflammation and benign hypertrophy).

What do these facts mean? Is there really an epidemic? Should men over 45 get biopsies? Do men over 40 need yearly PSA blood tests?

Question: Why was an herbal medicine (PC-SPES) that successfully treated both localized and metastatic prostate cancer removed by the FDA for "impurities" 7 years ago?

Question: Why are increasing numbers of men refusing prostate biopsies and turning to alternative forms of non-traditional therapies?

Question: Why does the 1940 textbook, *Neoplastic Diseases: A Treatise On Tumors* written by Dr. James Ewing, Professor of Oncology at Cornell University Medical Center, the most respected cancer pathologist of the 20th century, say: *Until recently carcinoma of the prostate was held to be a rare disease, forming 0.27% of the carcinomas in men....*

These poignant questions will be answered in the following pages, but one question remains that can be answered now: Is there a way to avoid biopsies? The answer to that question is a resounding "Yes," and comes from the international pioneer in prostate cancer imaging, Dr. Francois Cornud, Associate Professor of Interventional Radiology at Necker University Hospital in France.

In 1990 Dr. Cornud began using a new technology in Paris called color Doppler ultrasound which showed abnormal blood vessels in aggressive prostate cancers. His first textbook on this subject was published in French during 1993. A 2005 version by Dr. Olivier Helenon contains 1,424 pages of medical text using the latest diagnostic imaging methodologies. Textbooks by Dr. Cornud and Dr. Roy both appeared in 2006 on the updated version of the same topics. A French oncologist, Dr. C. Cuenod, commented at the 2003 International European Radiology Convention; "le degree de la neoangiogenese est correlee a l'agressivite tumorale au risque de metastases" translated, this means, the more vascular a tumor or the more blood vessels within it, the greater the risk of spread and metastases. This idea was repeated at the 2006 Journees Francaises de Radiologie with presentations by me and by investigators at the French Cancer Institute noting that 3D blood flow imaging correlates best with aggressive cancer diagnosis. The remainder of the subject matter in this book will cover new sonogram and MRI technologies that alter the fundamental nature of cancer diagnosis and offer elegant and rational advanced treatment options.

CHAPTER THREE

Rethinking Fundamental Knowledge

(A NEW FACT- BASED PERSPECTIVE ON CANCER)

"Una sola esperienza o concludente dimonstrazione…
basta a battere in terra questi ed altri centomila argomenti probabili"

"A SINGLE EXPERIENCE OR CONCLUSIVE DEMONSTRATION…IS
ENOUGH TO DEFEAT 100,000 POSSIBLE ARGUEMENTS"
–GALILEO GALILEI 16TH CENTURY

"Open your textbook to page 89 and *tear it out,*" said my Professor of Medicine in 1965. I could hardly believe my ears, however, I, and the entire second year class of '68 at the Upstate Medical Center of the State University of New York opened up our brand new pathology texts and tore out the page on inflammation. His words, "Medical knowledge is not perfect and knowledge is not a substitute for wisdom or experience" echoed in the lecture hall. "After all, blood letting was the medical standard for hundreds of years," he continued. My first awareness that medicine was an art as well as a science was born in that experience.

In 1986, I saw a young Irish woman and did a sonogram on her abdomen. This was unremarkable, and I asked her again why she was being examined. "Don't you remember me from two years ago? Don't you recall I was told I had three months to live back then?" she replied. I looked up her old chart and found pictures showing that she had wide-spread breast cancer that had metastasized to the liver, bones and abdominal glands at that time consistent with death within three to six months. "What did you do?" I asked. She answered, "I took vitamin

C and prayed." I repeated my ultrasound study confirming total absence of abdominal disease and learned from this encounter the certitude that alternative treatments had a potential role in modern medicine. Perhaps there was an art to various complementary therapies as well?

A similar awakening occurred in 1995 at a breast cancer conference hosted by New York University School of Medicine. The morning lecture by the famous Swedish mammography expert, Dr. Lazlo Tabar showed that a breast cancer measuring under 10 mm (^{1}/3 inch) in size had a 99 percent cure rate in five years by simply removing the tumor by a localized surgical lumpectomy. That afternoon, a chemotherapist of equal medical stature told the audience that chemotherapy and radiation treatments were routinely given for this type of cancer after surgical removal. The Swedish doctor jumped up and cried: "Didn't you hear my statistics this morning? What are you saying? No! What are you doing?"

I had a special reason for attending that conference. A dear friend had just been diagnosed with low grade breast cancer and asked me to search out new possibilities. Breast and prostate cancers have many clinical similarities since both are glands, and new breast cancer therapies may become potential prostate cancer treatments. As I heard the different opinions of the lecturers, I was concerned with the wide variety of "standards." For example, my friend had a frozen biopsy (immediate pathologic report) on her cancer at a university hospital in New York. In order to obtain optimum results, surgeons at Harvard wait three days for the specimen to be thoroughly prepared before using the microscope to review the biopsy material. After leaving the conference, I advised her that watching this slow growing cancer was a distinct possibility as well. She had her mastectomy the very next day. The fear of the potential negative predicted outcome had crippled her ability to make rational choices and reasoned decisions about alternative health options.

Five years ago physicians began questioning the value of bypass surgery for coronary artery disease. This led to more vigorous investigation of the mechanism of heart attacks. Dr. Eric Topol, an Interventional Cardiologist at the Cleveland Clinic, called into question the unchallenged idea that narrowing of the coronary arteries causes heart attacks. The culture of cardiology worldwide has been: fixing a narrowed artery to the heart will help the patient's heart do better. Traditional medicine has held the idea that coronary artery disease is akin to sludge building up in a pipe. Plaque (sludge) builds up over years and eventually clogs the artery causing a heart attack by blocking the blood supply to the heart. It was believed bypass surgery or angioplasty (using balloons to push back plaque in the arteries) would open the narrowed arteries and keep them from closing up completely. It was assumed this surgical intervention would prevent heart attacks.

Research from centers around the world has brought a new concept to light. The old idea that heart attacks occur from arteries narrowed by plaque is no longer the predominant model for therapy. Heart attacks occur when an area of plaque in the vessel wall bursts, causing a clot to develop over this region. It is the enlarging blood clot that blocks the artery. In up to 80% of cases, the plaque that suddenly erupts is not the one blocking the blood vessel. The dangerous plaque is soft, fragile and produces no symptoms. This region of diseased artery would not be seen by electrocardiograms, angiograms, stress tests or echocardiograms. These are silent killers now given voice by the ability to persistently review the unquestioned facts of medicine. New intra-arterial sonogram systems presented at the 2007 International Society of Endovascular Therapy Meeting are now able to detect these life threatening regions.

This finding explains the fact that most heart attacks occur at 4:00 a.m., when people are sleeping and not stressed. It explains the fact that most "coronaries" happen unexpectedly, without the warning of chest pain. For example, a jogger, the very picture of health, may run three miles effortlessly on one day and die of a heart attack the next. If a narrowed artery was the culprit, then the exercise of running would have produced "angina" or severe cardiac pains. Heart patients tend to have hundreds of vulnerable plaques. The rationale of unplugging one or two arteries no longer makes sense. Researchers are also finding that plaque and heart attack risk can change dramatically and quickly. Dr. Peter Libby of Harvard Medical School recently said, "The disease is more mutable than we thought." There has been much study on the role of inflammation producing the bursting of the arterial plaque. It has been theorized that the pivotal role of aspirin in preventing heart attacks may be as much due to its antiinflammatory properties as well as the proven anticlotting mechanism.

Years ago, my father, a still vigorous man and newly retired physician, was given only six months to live. At age eighty he developed mild abdominal pains after eating. His electrocardiogram was slightly abnormal. After he had his cardiac catheterization (dye study of the coronary heart arteries) he expected to be dismissed the next day. No one came to see him until a full two days after the procedure. The hospital cardiologists had reviewed it with several teams of doctors and finally told him that all his arteries were narrowed so badly that they had nothing to offer him other than the advice to get his affairs in order. I remember standing at his bedside, saying, "We'll find some way to help you, Dad" though, at that time I had no idea what it would be. I sent word of my father's problem to friends in and out of the medical community. A week later, a non physician friend brought me an article from the *New York Times* written by Dr. Dean Ornish revealing a vegetarian diet could reverse atherosclerosis (hardening of the artery). My father went on a strict diet and his coronary symptoms gradually subsided over the years.

At age 87, my father developed cancer of the bile ducts, a very slow growing form of tumor. Because he had been labeled with the diagnosis of end stage heart disease, curative surgery was not proposed, and he had stents (tubes) inserted into the bile duct to keep the tumor from blocking the flow of bile from the gallbladder to the digestive tract Because he did not have definite surgical removal of the very small initial tumor, the growth kept intermittently blocking the bile flow through the tubing. He would return to the hospital every three months to have the bile duct re-opened. Soon, he became depressed, as do so many patients with chronic diseases and the quality of life alterations that accompany endlessly ongoing treatments. One Sunday morning my mother called me saying, "Come quickly. I think your father is dying. He can't get out of bed." I rushed over to see him and found him barely responsive to my questions.

Finally, I shouted, "Get up! We are going for Sunday brunch at the country club. Put on your clothes." With a great deal of coaxing he dressed, got into the car and drove with us to the club. A small hill stretched between us from the parking lot to the dining room. "Dad," I said, "hold my arm and we'll walk up the hill together." He took one step, hesitated, then took another, hesitated again, and yet another. Halfway up the climb, he stopped—looked at me—smiled, and said, "You don't have to help me now. I can walk the rest of the way by myself." And he did. Six and a half years after he was supposed to succumb to his heart disease, he had beaten the odds and reversed most of the coronary arterial plaque. When he ultimately died from his cancer, he was no longer on heart medication. As a practicing traditional physician trained in radiology, I did not fully believe in miracles until it occurred in front of me with my own family. This incident was further nail in the coffin that medical "truths" are 100 percent valid.

While new ideas are not quickly recognized and change is often resisted, the journey of my father's illness from the grave to the country club had me realize that old notions tend to persist in today's medicine. Everyone needs to keep looking at the difficulties in bringing innovations and unorthodox treatments to the medical marketplace in the field of cancer. People who said the earth revolves around the sun were burned as heretics 600 years ago. This inherent resistance to progress serves as a template to see the struggle one might have in disseminating new concepts in cancer diagnosis and treatment. What would happen to the American Cancer Society if cancer was finally cured?

The changing picture of what works to prevent heart attacks and why, emerged only after years of research that initially was met with disbelief. In 1986, Dr. Greg Brown of the University of Washington in Seattle published a paper showing heart attacks occurred in areas of coronary arteries where there was too little plaque to use a stent or to use bypass surgery. He was derided by many cardiologists. Around that time Dr. Steven Nissen of the Cleveland Clinic started looking at patient's coronary arteries with a tiny ultrasound camera and proposed the idea that the "hard" plaque that obstructed arteries was not the plaque that caused heart attack. It was the "soft" plaque that was grew quickly and burst that eventually produced the fatal coronary thrombosis. He was also greeted with skepticism by his peers. In 1999, Dr. Waters from University of California received a similar reaction to his study of patients without chest pain referred for angioplasty. He found that patients who went on a cholesterol lowering diets had fewer heart attacks then those who had angioplasty (catheter opening of the arteries). Even worse was the finding by Dr. Topol who discovered that the procedure of placing a stent (tube that mechanically opens an area that is narrowed) in a patient's diseased arteries can actually cause minor heart attacks in about 4 percent of the patients. This adds up to a great deal of heart damage to people who chose a treatment to prevent it.

In the year 2004 a front-page article in the *Wall Street Journal* reported on the reasons that certain cancer therapies do not work under standard medical principles as well as expected. According to the report, there are "stem" cells that create invasiveness in cancers. These cells will keep dividing and growing while other less resistant cancer cells die off after a few growth periods. This may explain the phenomenon of cancers regressing under radiotherapy, chemotherapy or hormonal therapy only to return as more aggressive cancers later. This re-occurrence was common in men treated with the Chinese herb mixture that was marketed under the name PC-SPES (P=prostate, C=cancer and "spes" is the Latin word for HOPE). This non-traditional oriental concoction shrunk the prostate, reduced an elevated PSA test to negligible values and stopped not only the cancer but many times arrested growth of the metastatic disease as well. The existence of cancer stem cells also explains tumor recurrence after surgery where the margins are considered clean. In many medical series it has been shown, if vigorously sought, that tumor cells may be hiding in the postoperative site. Indeed, work by

Dr. Fred Lee, inventor of the ultrasound guided prostate biopsy, showed that about half of the clinically localized cancers have actually spread outside the prostate at surgery or by specialized diagnostic imaging scans.

When one realizes that a single cell missed by the microscope may eventually reform into an aggressive tumor, the rationale for curative surgery becomes unclear. Also defusing the need for immediate operative intervention is the observation that at least twenty-five percent of breast cancers and fifty percent of prostate cancers neither tend to grow nor metastasize. The question for the patient becomes not, "How should I treat this," but rather, "Should I do anything at all but monitor this from time to time?" This attitude is further bolstered by the growing awareness of an entity called "interval cancers" These rapidly growing tumors may arise spontaneously within months of a normal exam. The previous or ongoing treatment of a low grade tumor may give false hope to a patient who has just developed a high grade tumor and doesn't think he needs further observation. To further complicate matters, autopsy studies on men dying from automobile accidents in Boston demonstrated prostate cancers in some men in their 30's. More alarming is the knowledge many highly aggressive "interval cancers" do not cause PSA elevation and are mostly found in patients with low PSA levels.

Prostate cancers have similarities to breast cancers in many aspects, since both organs are glands. Autopsy data from a Harvard Medical school study of women dying from automobile accidents revealed thirty-nine percent of women between the ages of forty to fifty years had breast cancer cells when only 1 percent of women would have been expected by usual clinical standards to have breast tumors. A multicenter mammogram study twelve years ago on Long Island women, where the breast cancer incidence is disproportionately high, showed that biopsies for malignant appearing calcifications on x-ray mammography revealed a greater percentage of microscopic cancers not in the areas suspected of being cancer, but rather in the unsuspected regions adjacent to the expected cancer sites. Another Harvard study presented to the New York Cancer Society at the 2005 Annual Meeting showed data demonstrating the breast is continually developing benign and malignant tumors. Most of these never become clinically significant. The message from these reports is: *many cancers are not lethal.*

Half a century ago, pathologists found a high percentage of men without "clinical" prostate cancer to have malignant cells in the operative specimens of surgery for relief of benign prostatic obstruction. In the absence of demonstrable tumor invasion, perhaps cancer formation should be considered a non-threatening aspect of normal body aging, or at worst, a chronic disease.

Is there a way to determine whether a cancer is part of the natural aging process to be watched or whether the malignancy will have deadly consequences? In 1985, a prominent British physician, David Cosgrove, published a paper in the *American Journal of Radiology* demonstrating the presence of blood flows in breast cancers. After reading his article, I hopped on a plane and visited the Radiology Department at Hammersmith Hospital in London. There I observed the test first hand and envisioned future potential uses. I noted the new generation of sonogram equipment now had the capability to show pictures of blood vessels. The arteries and veins supplying a tumor could be clearly imaged. Moreover, the actual flowing blood in the cancer could be seen and velocity of flow of blood in the vessels accurately measured. At an international conference in Italy in 1997, Dr. Rodolfo Campani, an Italian radiologist specializing in studying the blood flows of cancers at the University of Pavia Medical Center, showed the criteria to differentiate malignant cancer vessels from benign tumor blood vessels. Benign vessels are few in number, smoothly outlined, follow straight courses and branch regularly. Malignant vessels are many in number, irregularly outlined, irregular in course and crooked in branching patterns. There are other blood velocity differences that are too technical for this book; however, it should be noted that malignant vessels have greater flow volumes at the end of the heart pumping cycle than benign vessels. These findings have been confirmed by other investigators at the 2006 World Congress of Interventional Oncology. Malignant blood vessels may be accurately and noninvasively detected by newer Doppler sonography techniques and advanced blood flow MRI protocols.

ULTRASOUND AND SONOGRAPHY

Sonar was invented by American industrialists for checking metal flaws in railroad ties. It was perfected by the US military for navigational use and under water scanning. Early medical uses included imaging disorders of the eye, heart and the developing fetus. As computers grew in sophistication, so did the applications of ultrasound, and now, it is often used as the first diagnostic test for many medical disorders. Doppler sonar created in 1972 gives pictures of flow movement in the human body in the same way it shows motion in the weather patterns (Doppler radar) that one sees on television weather reports. Doppler technology has been around for years. One patient told me that he designed and built missiles for the US Army at the White Sands Proving

Grounds in New Mexico in the 1950's. He related that the technique was so sensitive that it had to be modified continually and toned down considerably. Apparently, if an air conditioner was turned on a mile away, the missile's detection system would arm and prepare to fire. Indeed, one time a missile actually took off towards a moving train and followed it along the Santa Fe railroad tracks.

Urologists in Japan, oncologists in England, surgeons in the Netherlands, chemotherapists in Belgium, ultrasonographers in Norway and radiologists in France, seeing the success of sonograms in diagnosing malignant tumors in the breast, turned their attention to the study of the prostate. They concluded that the vascular pattern shown by the Doppler technique held the key to the degree of malignancy. Four years ago, German surgeons at the University of Ulm, the largest bone tumor center in Europe, showed bone cancers that were highly malignant had high blood flows. The current clinical use of Doppler equipment in Europe is keeping patients from unnecessarily losing their arms and legs. The standard treatment for bone cancer is amputation of the entire limb. Bone tumors that demonstrate no vascularity or low blood flows are now watched or treated more conservatively.

Dr. Nathalie Lassau, an interventional radiologist at the Institute de Cancerologie Gustav Roussy, an internationally known cancer center in Paris, published similar findings on the deadly skin cancer, melanoma. Her article in the *American Journal of Radiology* in 2002 revealed lethal skin cancers to be highly vascular and skin cancers that could be watched were not vascular. Dr. Lassau is currently investigating medicines to reduce blood flows to cancers in hope of lessening their malignant consequences and has presented this work at numerous international meetings. Her finding 3D Doppler sonography correlates best with the pathologic process was highlighted at the 2006 JFR Meeting in Paris. Newer MRI imaging protocols are currently being fine tuned based on the proven high accuracy of the Doppler sonography data.

The blood flow patterns depicted by Doppler sonography provide a way to quantitatively measure and serially monitor the severity of malignancy. Blood flow analysis can show which cancers are aggressive, since these have many vessels and which respond to treatment, since the size and number of tumor vessels decreases with successful therapies. Although this concept was described in the early 1990's in Europe, it was first mentioned in the American literature in 1996 at the American Roentgen Ray Society Annual Meeting. Dr. E. Louvar from Detroit,s Henry Ford Hospital combined radiology and pathology studies to determine that the power Doppler flows in malignancies was related to the vessels that fed aggressive tumors.

Why is this important? Significantly higher Gleason scores (more dangerous tumors described later) were seen in cancer biopsies of high Doppler flow areas compared to cancers with no Doppler flows. Dr. D. Downey at John Robarts Research Institute of the University Hospital in Ontario, Canada has looked at vascular imaging techniques and 3-dimensional imaging of blood vessels. Blood vessels can be rendered in 3-D with angiography (high intensity dye injected into arteries), CT scanning (medium intensity dye), MR angiography (low intensity dye), 3-D color Doppler imaging and 3-D power Doppler imaging. In this article published from the *American Journal of Radiology* in 1995, he noted that power Doppler was better able to delineate the abnormal vessel architecture than color Doppler techniques in prostate cancers.

A 2004 newsletter from the Prostate Cancer Research Institute reported that hormone therapy may change the way the pathologist interprets a cancer. Androgen deprivation therapy, (ADT) makes it more difficult to grade the tumor with the microscope. Men who have been on ADT should have a Doppler sonogram study to confirm the absence of residual disease. If there are areas of abnormal blood vessels, biopsy may be considered. Many patients who have been treated for cancer accept the presence of abnormal blood flows as proof of recurrence and choose treatments accordingly without further biopsies. Most patients use the amount of decrease in number of the visible blood vessels to represent the degree of success. Dr. Pam Unger, a prostate cancer pathology specialist at Mount Sinai Hospital in New York, mentioned in a personal communication that radiation changes also caused difficulties in reading the microscopic slides. Furthermore, pathologists generally don't look for blood vessels, and thus, do not routinely evaluate the vascular pattern in the specimens they interpret. Another problem with biopsy interpretation is the over-the-counter herbal medicine market. Many of the products for prostate health have some hormonal effects that shrink the prostate and improve symptoms. However, no one has determined if the pharmacologic properties of these alternative health treatments change the cells of the prostate to mimic cancer when the pathologist studies them under a glass slide. Today, one must also consider the possible toxic effects on the prostate of medicines and supplements made outside the US.

A 60 year old patient came to me who had been diagnosed via biopsy with high grade cancer. The biopsy was reviewed by several experts who agreed upon the serious nature of his problem. Unsatisfied, he had another urologist take a second biopsy, who confirmed his hopes that he indeed had a less malignant tumor. To settle the matter, he flew from southern California for clarification by the Doppler test. The use of the sonogram, though non-invasive, was invaluable in succinctly detecting the level of malignancy of the tumor. The blood flow sonogram showed the majority of the tumor to be low grade (without blood vessels), but a critically located region near the capsule was high grade (vascular) and was beginning to break through the capsule of the prostate where it could more easily metastasize. This was confirmed by MRI exam and later by surgery when the tumor was completely removed.

A 55 year old man came to me reluctantly because his biopsy was negative, but his PSA was steadily rising. He had the standard biopsy in which three biopsy samples are taken from each side of the midline of the gland, one each at the base, the mid-gland and the apex. The cancer was centered in the midline where the biopsy never reached.

Yet another 70 year old man was told he had a high grade cancer, upon seeing the sonogram demonstrating the tumor measured 4 mm (^{1}/8 inch) and was set away from the capsule of the prostate, he decided to watch it and see if it grew. Six months later it had not grown. Twelve months later showed no growth. Eighteen months later there was no change. He informed me that he is postponing his twenty four month follow up scan because he is now traveling around the world.

A 52 year old from the Midwest had a PSA of 5 one year ago. Thirty one biopsies failed to disclose any cancer. Upon his visit to our center, a large anterior non palpable mass was clearly visible. It had broken through the capsule by this time. Ironically, his latest PSA had lowered to 3. Back in Michigan, he was persuaded by his urologist to be rebiopsied. This time a Gleason 4+3 was discovered.

A 50 year old from the South was referred for local cryosurgery. He had 18 biopsies showing Gleason 4+4 on the left and was considering HIFU or focal cryosurgery to maintain his potency. All his biopsies on the right were benign. Upon digital rectal examination, I felt a mass on the right and told him so. "Doctor", he said, "the biopsy shows a tumor on the left, the right is normal" Upon seeing the large mass of abnormal blood vessels on the right and the penetration of the tumor through the right capsule and the comparatively few abnormal vessels on the left, he agreed to have an MRI exam. The special computerized MRI study confirmed bilateral tumors. He decided to try HIFU as a first line treatment as he and his young wife were intent upon expanding their family. They were relieved, however, that the tumor on the left was not as aggressive on the scans as the biopsy indicated and that they were chosing a bilateral treatment instead of a focal one-sided therapy.

CHAPTER FOUR
Practical Prostate Anatomy and Diagnosis

A very basic urologic anatomy will be presented at this juncture to highlight the strategic benefits of the newer technologies:

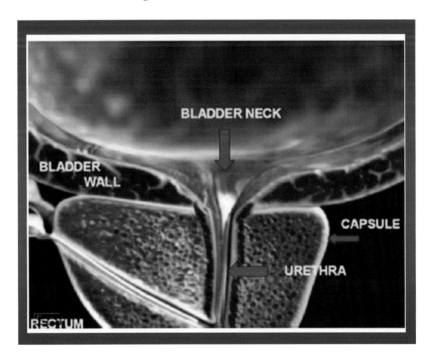

Fig. 4.1. Anatomy of prostate gland and capsule

Important anatomic zones are the base of the prostate which is next to the bladder, the apex which is farthest from the bladder and the midgland located between the base and the apex. Like an avocado, the gland has an outer zone called the peripheral zone in which most cancers occur and a central zone (similar to the avocado pit) where few cancers occur and the growths that develop are usually benign. The nerves that are necessary for erection lie along the gland on both right and left side of the exterior of the prostate capsule.

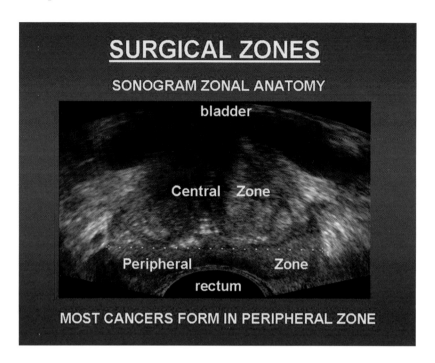

Fig. 4.2 Ultrasound anatomy of prostate

Gleason Grading Numbers and Prognosis

It is important to understand at the outset that biopsies may be random and sometimes difficult to interpret. Indeed, one of the reasons I attended the Armed Forces Institute of Pathology was to learn the discrepancy between what the microscopic analysis predicted and the actual outcome. It appears that the pathology reading is best correlated with the imaging findings on x-rays, CT, MRI, PET and ultrasound studies. This was particularly true in bone cancers, since the microscopic picture of a healing fracture is almost identical to a serious malignancy.

I remember Dr. Jack Rabinowitz, Chief of Radiology at my residency program at The Brooklyn Hospital (and later Chief of Radiology at Mount Sinai Medical Center in New York) in 1970 showing a surgeon that his working diagnosis of bone cancer was unsupported by the radiologic findings suggesting lymphoma (gland cancer) metastatic to the bone. The surgeon reviewed the case, decided against operating, and the patient was successfully treated medically instead.

Tumor grade refers to the microscopic appearance of cancer tissue obtained after biopsy or surgery and is named for the 1966 inventor, Dr. Donald Gleason. The Prostate Cancer Research Institute Newsletter of 2002 states only ten laboratories in the United States are accurate in their interpretation of the Gleason Score (GS or Gleason Sum) which determines the invasiveness of cancers. The Prostate Cancer Research Institute Newsletter of 2006 notes that pathologists have changed their grading patterns to higher numbers over the last decade and there is ongoing discussion of changing the methodology to more clearly represent significant disease. Indeed, pathologists have acknowledged that the numbers from biopsies are often upgraded or downgraded when the actual gland is surgically removed and examined by microscopic sections.

Tumor grading is defined as a property of cancer independent of tumor location found in either a biopsy or operative specimen. The GS primary grade is the most important pattern that the pathologist sees in the tumor under the microscope and must be greater than 50 percent of the total pattern. The secondary grade is the next most predominant pattern and must be at least 5 percent of the total pattern. The Gleason score is the sum of both patterns observed. Grades are from 1–5 with 5 being the most malignant and scores range from 2–10 with 10 being the most malignant. Newer investigation techniques used by modern pathologists are now showing that many cases of Gleason Sum=2 cancer were actually an abnormal benign growth (adenosis) which mimics cancers but is not actually malignant. In current practice, a Gleason 6 (3+3) or lower may be considered a low grade tumor while a higher number is often significantly more malignant.

While prognosis or survival is often correlated with Gleason score, perhaps a better indicator would be the response of a tumor's vascularity to the current treatment regimen. A study from the National Cancer Institute on this subject was presented by Dr. Lucia in the May 2005 issue of *The Journal of Urology*. This indicated that the high grade cancers (Gleason 8–10) induced by *finasteride* were limited to one side rather than both sides of the prostate gland. Clearly more research must focus on the controversial area of cancers being aggravated by prescription medications.

An international study by Dr. Yan Fong of Singapore and Professor Michael Marberger, Chief of Urology at the University Hospital of Vienna, Austria presented at the 100th American Urological Association 2005 Meeting discussed the effect of age on Gleason Scoring. In men under age 65 years, the accuracy of the initial needle biopsy was 22% when compared to the carefully reviewed radical prostatectomy surgical specimen in the pathology department. 64.6% of men younger than 65 had their Gleason Scores revised upwards to a more malignant tumor while 13.4% had their Gleason Scores revised downward. On a happier note, a Stanford University Medical Center study presented at the same meeting by Dr. K. Lee and colleagues showed that a positive family history of prostate cancer is not associated with worse outcomes after radical prostatectomy.

MRI OF THE PROSTATE

There are several MRI formats for examining the prostate. MRI routinely refers to the image of signal intensity in the gland with the patient in the tube of the unit. EC-MRI uses an endorectal coil (EC) to improve resolution in the prostate. S-MRI or spectroscopic MRI involves analysis of the chemical composition of the prostate tissues with emphasis on the compound *choline*. DCE (DYNAMIC CONTRAST ENHANCED)-MRI uses the injection of a contrast agent *gadolinium* that reveals the blood flow within tumorous prostatic tissue. 3.0 Tesla (higher strength) and CAD-CE-MRI also referred to as Full Time Point (FTP) CE-MRI will be discussed at length in the last chapter.

MRI shows cancer as a loss or decrease of the normal glandular prostatic tissue signal, however, other benign pathologies, such as calculi, hemorrhage (bleeding from recent biopsy), stones, BPH and inflammation, may also produce this effect. Some infiltrating types of cancer will not produce any visible changes. The 2007 data from University of California San Francisco shows a 78% sensitivity (few false negatives) and a 55% specificity (many false positives). MRI was originally used to stage the spread of cancer outside the prostate gland also denoted as ECE (extra capsular extension). UCSF data showed ECE high specificity (95%) but low sensitivity (38%).

EC-MRI using the endorectal coil inflated as a balloon was designed to better define the capsule of the gland and the seminal vesicles.

S-MRI was designed to detect intraglandular cancer and shows the aggression. The spectroscopic chemical analysis of cancer shows higher levels of choline and citrate than in normal prostatic tissues. The analysed sections of the prostate are divided into a grid pattern of such a size that small cancers could be missed. While this technique appeared useful for larger tumors, a 2005 *RADIOLOGY* article noted an overall sensitivity of 56% for tumor detection. Currently S-MRI is practiced at few medical centers in the US and is losing popularity at many international academic facilities. A 2006 presentation by Dr. O. Rouviere from Lyon, France at the French Radiology Meeting highlighted the problem that S-MRI was not effective in analyzing tumor extension into the fatty tissues adjacent to the prostate gland.

DCE-MRI is widely used and has improved specificity by about 80% according to the 2006 *RADIOLOGY* article by Drs. J. Futterer and J. Barentsz and sponsored by the Dutch Cancer Society. This group has developed a 3-D S-MRI system that improves the overall accuracy of standard S-MRI.

An MRI exam shows the extent of cancer but not the activity. In patients successfully treated by hormones, the abnormality may still persist on the MRI picture; whereas, the Doppler test has the advantage of showing the blood flows are greatly reduced or completely absent. Spectroscopic MRI, (widely known as S-MRI) also designed to show activity, has not been shown to be as sensitive as physicians had hoped. Indeed, one physician colleague, who flew from New York City to San Francisco for this test, was told the S-MRI showed extensive cancer, however, twelve biopsies revealed no cancer. At the 2004 meeting of the New York Roentgen Society devoted to Prostate Cancer, Dr. Steven Eberhardt, of Memorial Sloan Kettering Cancer Center, said that S-MRI was inaccurate in the presence of prostatitis because it produced false positive results. He went on to clarify the pro's and con's of regular MRI with the use of an endorectal coil mentioning that evaluation of the base is difficult due to the normal variation of anatomy of the prostate. Benign prostatic hypertrophy, commonly called BPH, often distorts the peripheral zone which is the most common site for cancer. Also, stones and hemorrhage (bleeding) from biopsies, and variations of the central prostatic zonal (internal) anatomy, could simulate cancers. Dr. Jelle O. Barentsz, Vice Chair of Research, at the University Medical Center Nijmegen, Netherlands, said that S-MRI results would be inaccurate following androgen deprivation therapy (hormone therapy, Chinese herbs, PC-Spes, etc) and disagreed that prostatitis was a problem. He also solved the problem of endorectal coil movement by injections (glucagons) to paralyze the colon for a full hour to complete the entire exam. One of my older patients, who had visited Dr. Barentsz in Holland, wryly observed that he did not have a normal bowel movement following the exam until 96 hours later. The consensus at the 2006 JFR Meeting was this: S-MRI would be discontinued in the future if the new generation of MRI units (3 Tesla with twice the strength of the standard 1.5 Tesla units) did not provide more accurate results.

Endorectal coils (EC) inserted into the rectum to afford close up views of the prostate gland have other difficulties observed since they tend to migrate upwards into the looser and wider part of the bowel rather than remain fixed where the prostate narrows the rectum. This results in degraded images of the apex (part of the prostate closer to the narrow anus). Physicians are now learning that pressure on the urinary bladder from the abdominal wall will deform the prostate, and they observe that the same occurs with the flattening of the rectal border of the prostate by the endorectal coil. Additionally, this tube is by itself uncomfortable, promoting more patient motion and degrading the exam results. The stiller the patient remains and quieter the patient's insides, the better the MRI images turn out. My practice has optimal results without using an endorectal coil as long as the CE-MRI is simultaneously compared with the sonographic findings. Lastly, the new non invasive treatments may cause dilation of the intraprostatic urethra or abnormal kinking and narrowing. This area is distorted by the pressure of the endorectal coil rendering diagnosis of these conditions more difficult.

Another problem with MRI exams is the variation of normal anatomy and the changes in the prostate formed by the commonplace benign enlargement called benign prostatic hypertrophy also known as benign prostatic hyperplasia (BPH). It has been widely acknowledged that the internal anatomy of the prostate may vary from individual to individual. It was becoming obvious that benign enlargement made MRI exams more difficult for physicians in this field to interpret. However, it was assumed that the capsule of tissue that held and contained the gland and also prevented spread of the tumor to regions outside the prostate was regular. It was shown in 2004 in the *American Journal of Radiology* that there is a normal irregularity to the capsule of the prostate in about 10% of men. This is surprising news to the imaging medical community and deserves further study. Unfortunately, the finding of capsular irregularity has been one of the cardinal signs for spread of the cancer in the prostate.

In diagnosing tumors physicians look for a dominant mass, a tumor bulge and loss of the normal internal prostatic architecture (usually in the peripheral zone). At the 2004 New York Roentgen Society Annual Conference a new use for the MRI was suggested to solve the problem of the frequent misplacement of radio-therapy fields due to the great variability of the prostatic anatomy in the base and the apex. MRI planning would provide the radiotherapist with a better volume rendering of the prostate so that the radiation may be more effectively targeted. At the 2004 meeting of the American Roentgen Ray Society's 104th Annual Meeting, the Director of MRI at the Mayo Clinic, Dr. Catherine Roberts, said that both MRI and radioactive isotope scans overdiagnose metastatic disease to the bones. In fact, one of my younger patients with prostatic inflammation had an MRI demonstrating no tumor in the prostate but markedly abnormal pelvic boney images. After the studies were reviewed by the radiologists at several specialty orthopedic centers in New York, agreement was reached that the suspicious areas needed biopsy results to ensure that there was no malignancy. Multiple biopsies showed no cancer. The changes were postulated as a side effect to calcium building hormones. Another young man had a small prostatic abnormality and multiple boney malignant findings. This non smoker had a rare type of lung cancer that had diffusely spread to the bones and the prostate.

Furthermore, many high grade prostate cancers have low PSA levels because they do not produce PSA secretions. The 2004 International Congress of Radiology in Montreal noted that only 15 percent of urologists use any form of MRI to evaluate the prostate and that use is generally to see if the tumor has spread to the adjacent glands. Researchers at the International BPH Forum in San Antonio in 2005 postulated that MRI would be more effective if the glands's hypertrophy was reduced. Indeed, Dr. H. Mao, a radiologist at the Emory University in Atlanta, suggested, in the 2005 issue of *Diagnostic Imaging,* that the latest version of the MRI (called 3T MRI) is not only useful for monitoring and staging prostate cancer, but "would recommend it for screening if it could be comfortable and affordable, since it shows the prostate structure so clearly." The initial experience in using MRI and S-MRI in finding cancer recurrences after radiation therapy was published in *Radiology* August 2005 by Dr. Pucar from Memorial Cancer Center. This is an important study since 25% of all patients that receive a diagnosis of prostate cancer are treated with external beam radiation therapy. The recurrence rate or relapse of tumor after 5 years is 15% for low risk patients and 67% for high risk patients. The results show that MRI, sextant biopsy and digital exam each had 90% specificity, but S-MRI had a lower specificity than these at 78%. Apparently the treated benign gland may simulate a cancer leading to false positive results. A 2006 article in *American Journal of Radiology,* by Dr. Wetter and colleagues, noted MRI spectroscopy did not significantly add more information than regular MRI when compared to the surgical specimens.

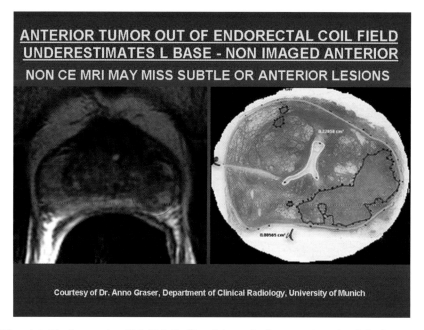

Fig. 4.3 Endorectal coil MRI (left) with pathology section (right) showing full extent of tumor

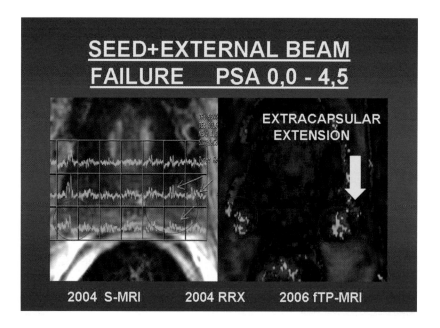

Fig. 4.4 Spectroscopic MRI (left) and dynamic contrast computerized MRI (right) showing tumor extending outside the prostate capsule (arrow)

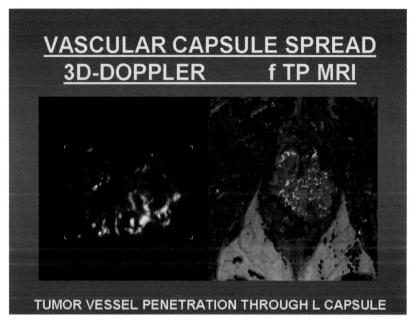

Fig. 4.5 Doppler sonogram of abnormal vessels (left)
Vascular MRI showing tumor (right)

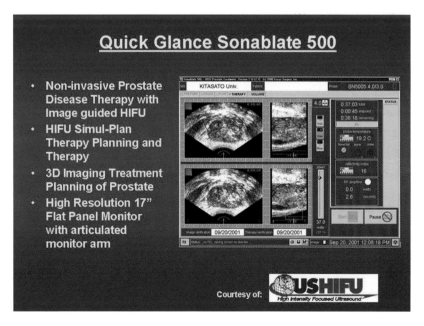

Fig. 4.6 Aggressive tumor (red) appeared within 7 months

SONOGRAPHY OF THE PROSTATE

I started examining the prostate thirty-four years ago with equipment that took sonograms from the skin surface on the lower part of the abdomen over a full urinary bladder. These were termed "transabdominal" pelvic sonograms. Fifteen years ago, probes were developed to insert into the rectum providing better images by placing the tip closer to the prostate. This study was called "transrectal" ultrasound or TRUS.

Twelve years ago I worked with urologists performing prostate biopsies under ultrasound guidance. I would scan the prostate and tell the surgeon the suspicious area to biopsy. The Doppler blood flows have proven to be the best indicator of highly malignant tumors as a region of high flow is 450% more likely to have a positive biopsy result. The American College of Radiology uses the blood flow density as an indicator for the best area to biopsy, as stated in the 2004 edition of *The Standards of the American College of Radiology*. Five years ago, the Austrians perfected 3-D imaging of the prostate which allowed physicians to optimally visualize the outer capsule of the prostate. This is a particularly important border since the spread of cancer outside the capsule means it is no longer operable. At the International Congress of Radiology in 2004, Dr. David Cosgrove, a leading English authority of color and power Doppler ultrasound imaging, voiced his approval of the use of this technology to determine the aggressiveness of prostate cancers.

While many men may be reluctant to avail themselves of current modalities detecting cancer in the prostate, an exam may ease the mind of a patient who may believe he has cause for concern, and allay some unnecessary, even irrational fears. A negative test alone would provide a significant comfort zone due to its high accuracy. A positive test that shows no blood flow means that a tumor is of a less aggressive nature, indicating that it will grow slowly. This is critically useful knowledge for men choosing watchful waiting or alternative treatments. The prostate sonogram is simple because it requires no preparation. It is safe as there are no x-rays or needles. It is fast since the technology is computerized. It is painless due to the non-invasive nature of the technology. It is only minimally uncomfortable since the small lubricated probe inserted into the rectum has a wide field of view so that little movement of the device is required by the examining physician to scan all pertinent areas.

Concerned about the uncertainties of PSA levels and the potential threat of slow growing cancers, physicians and patients all too frequently opt to remove the entire prostate gland as a precaution. Now, according to a 2004 article by Dr. Thomas Stamey of Stanford University in California, a study conducted by researchers at Stanford have concluded that a full 98 percent of all prostates removed at Stanford over the past five years were removed unnecessarily. Only 2 percent warranted removal due to cancers large enough to cause concern. This surprising result falls on the heels of other findings by Dr. Stamey; for example, the elevated blood levels of an enzyme called prostate specific antigen, or PSA, is a natural occurrence in men as they age, and not a definitive mark of a cancerous growth. Though men with aggressive cancers do indeed exhibit elevated levels of PSA, mild elevation of this enzyme is natural and, as Dr. Stamey explained, almost always related to normal enlargement of the organ as the aging process in men continues.

Dr. Stamey is the physician who pioneered the use of PSA to diagnose prostate cancer; so, his statement on its use is significant, as he is rethinking the use of PSA readings when considering options for cancer treatments. While PSA elevations are normal with age, any PSA blood test above ten is a reason for a biopsy. However, Dr. Stamey's team of researchers is looking for a more accurate way to determine the presence and severity of cancer in the prostate. Currently, they are working on a blood test that relates to the size of the tumor, but as yet, have met with little success. Remember, the most virulent cancers (called *anaplastic* tumors) do not make sufficient PSA to reflect in elevated values. This means the worst malignancies may have the lowest PSA numbers. This also means the more accurate sonogram technology may be used to replace this blood test.

When I first visited Dr. Cornud's clinic in Paris, I was surprised to see a younger man having his prostate scanned. He had been brought in by his wife. The wife's brother, in his late forties, had felt confident with his low PSA level and ignored concerns about the nodule his physician felt in his prostate. When he finally consented to a biopsy, the tumor had already spread to the bones. This dedicated woman was not going to let the same fate befall her husband. Another 40 year old man was referred in by his young wife when their infertility specialist had felt some "scarring of the prostate due to chronic infection." He had not had a PSA due to his youth and had a rubbery feeling gland on rectal probing which was compatible with infection. His sonogram showed a minor amount of scar formation and a major amount of highly aggressive tumor that had calcified in small clumps and felt more like firm scar tissue rather than rock hard cancer.

In the absence of a perfect modality for detecting cancerous cells in the prostate, there are standard tests for diagnosing prostate cancer. The digital rectal exam (DRE) uses the examiner's finger to find hard regions in the gland. Firm areas that are nodular and irregular usually indicate moderately advanced cancer. However, scarring of the prostate, tuberculosis (TB), sarcoidosis (glandular disorder like TB) and stones in this organ may simulate a tumor to palpation. This exam only checks the outside of the prostate and could miss growths on the side and in the deeper (anterior) regions that lie distant and out of reach of the probing examiner's finger.

The PSA blood test has been widely used for twenty years of screening men for cancer. A large study from Boston five years ago showed that the test underestimated the presence of cancer in two thirds of those examined and overestimated the likelihood of cancer in two thirds of the patients. Explanations that erroneous levels are due to prostatitis, or a previous biopsy, or a large gland, or inflammation or even a recent ejaculation are useful only in theory. A 2004 report from the Memorial Sloan Kettering Cancer Center, published in the prestigious *Journal of the American Medical Association,* reported that a man's PSA levels fluctuate naturally over time, which leads to false elevated scores. Dr. William Pitts, in an article in the 2003 *British Journal of Urology,* feels that the only use of PSA is to show recurrent tumors in the postoperative prostate. A measurable and rising PSA reading in a man with an irradiated or surgically removed prostate probably indicates a new malignancy in the post radiated or post surgical area or in the adjacent glands and bones. As more experience is gained with post operative patients using combined MRI and ultrasound scans, physicians are finding that patients without local recurrence may still have measurable PSA levels that in part, may be due to the spread of cancer to distant sites or may be due to inherent inaccuracies in the test itself. Many physicians still believe that a slowly and steadily rising PSA level indicates a true malignancy. To add to the controversy, an article published in the May 2004 issue of *The New England Journal of Medicine* reports that as many as 15 percent of men with normal PSA levels, less than four (normal 0–4 ng/ml) had cancer when assessed with biopsies. The study, conducted by Dr. Ian Thompson at the University of Texas Health Science Center in San Antonio, involved 2,940 men aged 62–79.

Dr. Len Lichtenfeld, Deputy Chief Medical Officer at the American Cancer Society responded to the article saying there "…are no easy answers about men with a low PSA level. They should have a biopsy. Cancers in such men are microscopic, a doctor cannot feel them, and there are no symptoms." He added, "We will find more prostate cancer, and we will find more cancers that didn't need to be found. We will cause some men harm that they didn't need to have." Dr. Gilbert Welch, a professor of medicine at the Department of Veteran's Affairs commented that this study should make men reconsider whether they want a PSA test at all. He said, "It is becoming increasingly clear that the more pathologists look for cancer, the more they will find it, but that does not mean the cancer is worth finding."

Although the sonogram test of the prostate may take different forms, all use ultrasound high frequency waves and sophisticated computer analysis. Using harmless sound waves ensures that the test is safe. The exam is rapid because of high technology imaging products. The study is accurate employing state-of-the-art computer reconstruction. Generally, the probe is placed inside the rectum, although it may be applied to the perineum (area between the penis and anus) to obtain images if the rectal approach is not possible. The ultrasonographic physician or specially trained imaging technician looks at the instantaneous video appearing on the screen, taking pictures and measuring images according to a standard protocol, and notes and documents abnormalities. Two dimensional pictures are taken in "real time" which are similar to the images of the inside the pregnant mother's womb showing moving babies or the fetal heart beating. The 3-D or three dimensional technology that shows the face of the baby is now being successfully applied to the prostate. It is different, as it is faster, yet contains more information than the standard 2-D sonogram. Essentially, the 3-D machine takes a volume of pictures and stores this data inside the unit's computer banks. The data may be analyzed immediately or later reviewed and reconstructed in various angles or planes. In comparing 2-D with 3-D imaging, one can say the sonographer looks and then takes pictures with the 2-D system; whereas, with the 3-D technology pictures are taken which are then looked at and formally evaluated later. If a significant problem is seen and annotated with the 2-D exam, it cannot be later observed except by completely re-scanning the patient. The 3-D rendition may be reviewed over and over without recalling and re-examining the patient. 3-D imaging has made exam time shorter providing more patient comfort. The images are then analysed on a special computer work station allowing optimal rendering of the prostate in multiple planes as required.

An important variation of the 3-D is called 4-D, which adds the element of time to the exam and is used for the advanced treatments described later in this book. While the 3-D sonogram takes only minutes to perform, 25 volume scans are performed every second in 3-D planes resulting in about 1,000 images that need to be reviewed and interpreted. Of the many technical features of 3-D imaging, "automatic acquisition" makes this test equivalent to an MRI or CT scan of the prostate, as it is multi-planar (in 3 planes) and accurately reproducible for comparison with an earlier or later study. The probe doesn't move inside the patient. The electronic array inside the probe sweeps back and forth, like a fan, over the prostate gland. A set of raw electronic data is stored in the sonogram memory that can be manipulated and studied as required at any time. The primary diagnostic breakthrough of 3-D/4-D imaging is to show slices of the prostate that see the capsule (outer margins) in what is called a coronal view.

This special view, available only on 3-D equipment, allows one to see invasion of cancer more easily. Specifically, the spread of cancer outside the prostate gland or extra-capsular extension is well seen with this technique. This is critical clinical information of tumor outside the capsule changes the cancer from operable to inoperable. The patient's own vascular pattern that determines aggression can be overlaid on the 3-D scan, which adds greatly to the assessment of the disease and the feasibility of treatment possibilities. This is notably useful in men with low grade cancers who wish to be followed with watchful waiting or alternative therapies thereby avoiding surgery or radiation. Most low grade tumors remain localized and may be watched or controlled with non invasive or minimally invasive treatments. The standard MRI cannot demonstrate tumor aggression in the moment, although comparison from previous exams show progress and interval changes.

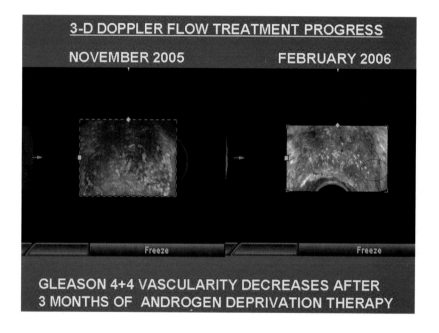

Fig. 4.7 3-D Doppler sonogram showing diminution of red vessels after treatment

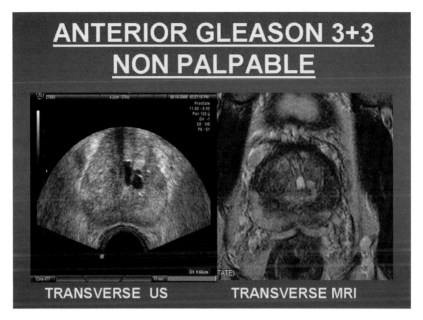

Fig. 4.8 Tumor in front of prostate cannot be felt by finger on back of prostate

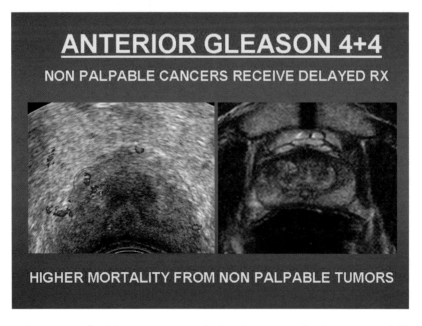

Fig. 4.9 Non palpable tumors spread silently since early diagnosis is difficult

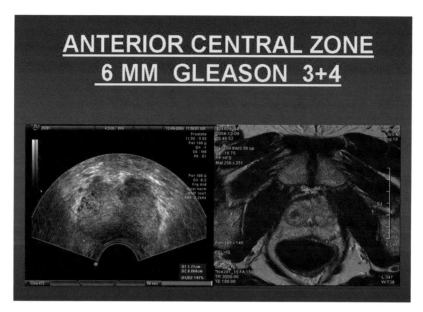

Fig. 4.10 Small tumors may be biopsied accurately under ultrasound or MRI guidance

Dr. Deborah Rubens, Associate Chair of Radiology and Surgery at the University of Rochester Medical Center, said in the January 2005 edition of *Diagnostic Imaging*, "With volume imaging, you're assured of getting everything you need. It standardizes exams, while providing us with new information and a new way to look at things." Dr. Rubens added that volumetric imaging is especially helpful when looking for multiple tumors or nodules. Since each region must be measured in several planes, it is easy to lose track of which nodule is which. She says that, "If you have them in a volume, you can just scroll through it. The next time that person comes in, it's easy to compare each problem area to what it looked like in the previous visit."

For example, Bob R, a 65 year old man from California had treated his Gleason 3+3 (low grade) tumor by macrobiotic lifestyle and naturopathic remedies that successfully controlled the cancer for five years. He was monitored in my office every six months, and there was no interval change demonstrated. On his 11th semiannual check up, I felt a firm mass on the digital rectal exam. The color flashed red on the computer screen, and we saw abnormal vessels. The 3-D PDS (3D power Doppler sonography) imaging showed the blood vessels penetrating through the capsule. The MRI exam later that day confirmed a large area of low grade cancer (Gleason 3+3) which remained unchanged and had not broken out of the prostate. However, where the new blood vessels appeared on the sonogram, the MRI revealed that there was a rupture in the capsule and new tumor penetration outside the prostate. After his initial disappointment, he realized that this red flag had probably saved his life by demonstrating a fresh and probably different type of cancer than the low grade tumor he had successfully treated for years with herbal supplements. He left our office a sobered but grateful person. Medical practitioners are realizing that the new entity called "interval cancers" appear more dangerous than the known cancers in both men and women. In this patient's case, a six month screening paid off as he knew he had alternate treatment options to choose. Dr. Robert Knapp, Professor Emeritus at Harvard Medical School and inventor of the CA125 blood test for cancer detection, described "interval cancers as the most virulent of prostate cancers that typically show up between screening examinations."

SCREENING TECHNOLOGIES

One must look at existing cancer screening technologies and results to determine if significant disease in adults is conclusively demonstrated. When I was a resident in training in 1970, everyone sought a yearly chest x ray. Routine chest x-rays were eventually phased out because the yield of a true clinical problem was extraordinarily low. *The Journal of the American Medical Association* in January 2004 noted that 38 percent of asymptomatic screened adults experienced false positive findings, and half of those with abnormal results found the experience "very scary"

Regarding lung cancer CT screening, the *Annals of Internal Medicine* in May 2004 showed that early cancers were detected at a greater rate than expected without this modality—evidence that screening decreased mortality was lacking. Total body CT cancer screening has been in vogue for years. The journal *RADIOLOGY* in 2004 alerted patients to the possibility of cancer causation by the x-ray dosage, due to the accumulation of excessive radiation in the body. A single screening exam at age 45 might be expected to cause a fatal cancer in 1 per 1,250 screened people. The incidence of new fatal cancer causation by regular annual screening for 30 years was estimated to be 1 per 50 screened people. In 2004, the US Preventive Services Task Force (USPSTF) endorsed colorectal, cervical and breast cancer screening. It did not endorse screening for coronary heart disease in low risk people. The USPSTF cited harms from false reassurance and injury incurred from subsequent invasive testing needed to clarify false positive results. A 2005 study by Dr. G. Scott Gazelle of the Massachusetts General Hospital Institute for Technology Assessment and Associate Professor of Radiology at Harvard Medical School, found whole body CT screening was not cost effective. Furthermore, he found that for every 1,000 patients screened, an average of 908 would have at least one false positive test result.

In my practice of screening men for prostate cancer with sonograms, my colleagues and I have been surprised to find about 5 percent of men with normal PSA had non-palpable aggressive cancers missed by clinical palpation. Now that sonogram screening for breast cancer has become as routine as the mammogram for women, it is logical to think that a non-invasive sonogram prostate screening modality may supplant the currently used PSA and digital rectal exams.

Perhaps this will be named similar to the woman's mammogram and be called the men's screening "prostagram" or "prostasound." In defense of the digital rectal exam (DRE) a presentation by Dr. J. Slaton, at the 100th American Urological Association Annual Meeting, 2005, noted that the digital rectal exam was more accurate in detecting high grade cancers than the PSA. In a series of 3817 patients, it was determined that the most highly aggressive tumors generated low amounts of PSA. Patients with a normal PSA and abnormal DRE had a 33% risk of high grade disease while patients with abnormal PSA and abnormal DRE had a 21% risk of high grade malignancy. He concluded saying, the "DRE continues to play a critical role in identifying patients with high grade cancer whose tumor is so poorly differentiated that it under produces relative low amounts of PSA."

There are possible errors with sonogram investigations. The regular 2-D sonogram may miss low grade cancers that have the same appearance as the normal gland, which account for up to 40% of prostate tumors according to Dr. D. Downey, in the 1997 journal *UROLOGY*. The overall accuracy is about 50 percent. The accuracy is better in glands that have never been subjected to a biopsy or treated in any way. The accuracy is lower in prostates that have been biopsied multiple times or in persons who have been treated with radiation or hormones. The power Doppler study adds about 30 percent more accuracy, since the abnormal blood vessels provide a road map to the tumor, however, detours on the road may occur in the presence of stones or calculi. Indeed, a US patent, number 5,860,929, was obtained by Norwegian scientists to determine power Doppler blood flows in optimally diagnosing prostate cancers. When a stone is identifiable, the sound waves bounce back so strongly that they create a false color pattern. This pattern to the trained clinician will not be mistaken for a tumor vessel. Fortunately, the Doppler technology has other formats that correctly identify the artifactual or spurious colors, distinguishing it from a true cancer. In my practice combining 3D PDS with focused computer aided vascular MRI exams, we have achieved a 97% overall accuracy in diagnosing and staging prostate cancers. An important exception occurs in the seminal vesicles, which sit on top of the prostate gland generating the fluid that produces the ejaculation. Early cancer spread to these paired vesicles may be missed by the 3D PDS. When a tumor is found near or adjacent to the seminal vesicles at the base of the prostate, MRI scans are mandatory.

Japanese investigators, Osamu Ukimura and Tsuneharu Miki, studied the use of 3D PDS in nerve sparing surgery, and presented their findings at the 2005 American Urological Association Meeting. Using European ultrasound systems during laparoscopic radical prostatectomy (LRP or robot guided surgical removal of the prostate) they were able to visualize the nerves of the prostate and protect them during surgery. This improved outcomes in terms of potency and continence. It also improved surgical margins meaning less volume of tumor was left behind. The real time imaging also showed the surgeon unsuspected tumors that were outside the planned operative field in 44 % of patients in the study. This alerted the surgeon to make a wider incision to include the newly discovered tumor. The authors also noted that injury to the adjacent rectal wall and bladder neck was avoided since these areas were continuously monitored. They concluded, "Real time TRUS during LRP can map important periprostatic structures and any clinically significant cancer nodules, potentially enhancing the precision of the laparoscopic procedure."

Another potential arena in which 3-D PDS is useful is the diagnosis and treatment of boney metastases. According to Dr. S. Paik, quoted in the 2005 *American Journal of Radiology*, malignant bone disease appears as a single focus 7 percent of the time. Among patients with a primary cancer, only 17 percent of rib disease shown on the nuclear isotope scan turns out to be truly malignant. In older patients rib fractures may be produced by coughing, strenuous exercise and non-recalled injuries. The use of high resolution sonography has proven 94 percent accurate in distinguishing between fractures and metastatic disease. Vascular prostate tumors may have vascular rib metastatic lesions. This feature of abnormal blood vessels is useful in following the regression of the tumor by the disappearance of the abnormal arteries and veins on the Doppler analysis by such treatments as radiation therapy or by radiofrequency ablation (RFA). Not surprisingly, the same article shows that state-of-the-art ultrasound detects ten times (10X) as many rib fractures as routine x-rays.

CHAPTER FIVE

Systematic Evaluation of Prostate Cancer Therapy

Before exploring newer technologies, let's review the various options in prostate cancer therapy:

STANDARD TREATMENTS
- Orchiectomy (surgical castration by removal of testes reducing male testosterone)
- Hormone therapies:
    (medical castration) Androgen Deprivation Therapy (ADT)
    Hormone Deprivation Therapy (HDT)
    Androgen Ablation Therapy (AAT)
    Androgen Suppression Therapy (AST)
    (Casodex, Lupron, Zolodex, DES)
- Watchful waiting
- Radical surgery
- External beam radiation
- Internal radioactive pellets (seeds)
- Cryosurgery (freezing)
- Radio Frequency Ablation (RFA) (heating metastatic tumors with radio waves)

ALTERNATIVE TREATMENTS
Dietary
Herbal (including products like PC-Spes) (also called Phytotherapy)
Radio Frequency Ablation (new use for heating a prostate tumor)
Radioactive particle embolization
Chemoembolization (shooting chemotherapy particles into the tumor)

- Alcohol and acetic acid injections
- Humanized monoclonal antibody (gene therapy)
- Stent obstruction (balloon blocking artery)
- Microsphere embolization (tiny particles clogging artery)
- Microwave heat denaturization
- Laser tissue destruction (heat)
- High Intensity Focused Ultrasound (HIFU) (heat)
- Antiangiogenic drugs (block new tumor blood vessels, like thalidomide)
- Genetic therapy (gene manipulation)
- Photodynamic therapy (light activating intraprostatic sensitizing agents)
- Magnets (mechanism unknown)
- Irreversible Electroporation (non thermal electromagnetic wave cellular destruction)
- Galvanotherapy (GT) or Electrochemotherapy (ECT)

In 1996, Dr. Michael Schachter, a prominent alternative medicine practitioner called me and asked me if I would like to learn a new treatment protocol for my patients. This new treatment was from a patient who had successfully regressed his own cancer. Dr. Schachter told me that he had developed his own effective alternative medical therapy protocols based on experience gained from the successes and failures of his own patients. Dr. Schachter introduced me to Larry Clapp who convinced me that his naturopathic healing had worked. When Larry allowed me to scan his biopsy proven high grade Gleason tumor, I saw all that remained was a scar. This meant a healed, inactive area had taken the place of a deadly cancer. When Larry told me that cancer was not a disease but a reactive response to a body disturbed by toxins and hormonal imbalance, I began to listen. As a formally trained radiologist, the thought of cancer not being *de facto* a disease didn't make sense; however, I was faced with the incontrovertible fact of a malignancy killed without drugs, radiation or surgery. As a physician trained in traditional medicine, this observation made me take serious notice. Since then, I have listened to my patients carefully and garnered experience with a wide collection of non-standard treatments. While I have seen every type of treatment have efficacy, I noted that some may work for some patients and not be helpful for others. Indeed, a successful treatment for a man with a low grade cancer may be useless when a new and different high grade tumor begins separate from the original and controlled disease. We are also learning that the bacteria in the stomach and intestines vary widely in people. This affects the way oral medications are absorbed by the body. The same is true of the acidity balances in the stomach and small intestine. There are ways to re-establish the normal values in the gastrointestinal tract and the reader is advised to investigate this area if oral preparations are not working as expected.

A gentleman from Virginia was seeing me every three months to evaluate his tumor. Four times a year he would try a different alternative treatment. I would confirm the beneficial effect for him on each of his visits. On a subsequent appointment I noted a high grade vascular prostate tumor that started invading his bladder on the left side. He went overseas for intense herbal and immune system treatments. Upon his quarterly return, the left side was inactive but the right side of the prostate gland with low grade cancer had now become aggressive and invaded the right side of the bladder. Finally, he found a regimen that controlled his tumors for the time being. My patients have taught me much and I acknowledge them for their courage in self healing. As long as I can continue to keep an open mind, I will be able to effectively explore, develop and share new healing modalities.

The approach I am suggesting is also based on thirty-four years experience in the field of diagnostic ultrasound, ten years of imaging the prostate with power Doppler blood flows and three years of performing 3-D power Doppler sonograms (3-D PDS) and comparing my results with high resolution MRI scans of the pelvis with special sequences formulated specifically for the prostate. I have diagnosed, observed and shared in the treatment of some 3,900 patients. Two men have died from their prostate cancer in this ten year time period. One young man, 42 years old, could not be saved by any type of conventional or unconventional treatment due to the virulent malignancy that raced uncontrolled by all efforts through his body. Another 69 year old corporate executive was in such denial that he refused to believe he had highly aggressive cancer for 11 months following my diagnosis. He flew in from Los Angeles twice a year for 4 years until I felt a nodule and showed him a new tumor. Each month he would call me and ask, "Could it be an infection? Could it be from an old injury? Could my weekly prostate massage have caused this? What about my foreign travel exposures? Could riding my bicycle on very bumpy roads produce this?" After a year of questions, to which I could only reply, "It is possible, but I strongly advise immediate definitive treatment." the malignancy finally blocked his bladder. He could no longer urinate which is a very late sign of widespread cancer. When a biopsy was performed, it showed a Gleason 5+4 (highly malignant), and he succumbed a year later.

My evaluations and recommendations are based on personal experience as well as practical knowledge in the field of medicine. In 1972, I asked my colleague, Dr.

Smith, the senior ultrasound physician at Harvard Medical School, where had he trained in the fledgling field of diagnostic ultrasound? He referred me to Dr. Hans Holm, Professor of Urology at the Gentofte Hospital outside of Copenhagen, Denmark. I left New York and went to study with Dr. Holm and his staff. Not only did I learn more about sonography, I also experienced aspects of medicine that were unfathomable by American standards. Specifically, kidney, liver and pancreatic tumors were being localized, and biopsies were taken with ultrasound guidance. American surgeons were taught at that time and are still cautioned today that biopsies of the pancreas are to be avoided at all costs because puncturing the pancreas will leak deadly digestive enzymes producing life threatening peritonitis (inflammation of the lining of the abdominal cavity). During my first week at this Danish teaching hospital and medical center I saw many biopsies of the kidneys and liver without complications. At the end of that week, a Danish fisherman required a pancreatic biopsy for a mass located in the upper abdomen. In those days the surgeons performed the sonograms in Denmark rather than the radiologists. Dr. Holm numbed the skin of the abdomen, put an 8 inch long needle into the pancreas under ultrasound guidance while the locally anesthetized patient was still awake and removed a core of tissue. Then, the lower level surgeons repeated the procedure, as did the Danish medical residents in training and finally myself. On morning rounds at 7:00 a.m. the next day, the patient who had no less than 32 biopsies of his pancreas, was complaining that he didn't like the clear liquid breakfast he was served-he wanted real food.

Twenty two years ago, my father, then a practicing physician, had one of the first PSA tests. It was 14, very much above the 4 ng/ml level that strongly indicated cancer. My sonogram on his prostate showed nothing suspicious. He never had a PSA exam again and never developed clinical prostate cancer. Ten years ago I had a PSA exam taken as part of a routine physical. It measured 22 ng/ml. This is extremely elevated-over 550 percent above the normal value. I had just started performing power Doppler sonograms and did one on myself. There was no abnormality. I now refuse to have the PSA exam performed on myself. Eight years ago the Director of the National Cancer Institute of Australia refused to endorse PSA tests. He publicly stated that the cure was worse than the disease. He kept his personal prostate philosophy and lost his job.

When I attended the major radiology conference in Europe in Paris, called Journees Francaise de Radiologie, (JFR2003) in October 2003, I used the 3-D technology for imaging the prostate that also gave holographic reconstructions of the capsule and vasculature of the gland. I had brought patients with me who had a biopsy proven tumors that I tested on the newer European and Japanese ultrasound units not yet available in the United States. I chose a European designed unit that had a specific probe for dedicated prostate scanning. Although the probe was in clinical use all over the world and even approved by the FDA in the United States, in particular, there was not one being used in North America for prostate cancer diagnosis. As of this writing, according to the manufacturer, I am one of the few physicians using the European designed Kretz ultrahigh resolution automated 3-D power Doppler system in the Americas for prostate diagnosis and treatment. Remarkably, the reason is urologists use the sonogram primarily to guide the prostate needle biopsy. This is done to sample an abnormality and avoid penetrating the bladder or bowel during the procedure. Radiologists do not see patients for this type of exam, since they are not referred out by the urologists. Patients do not ask for a radiologist when they have prostate problems. My intention is to inform patients about advanced international medical diagnostic modalities and offer new treatment options. This led me to change my profession from diagnostic radiologist to interventional radiologist where I tailor treatment to the patient based on newer concepts in radiologic imaging and maintain sensitivity to the patient's lifestyle choices regarding therapy. I have been inspired by my patients to do more than give diagnoses and recommend possible treatment choices. I work with the patient's team of urologist, internist, chemotherapist and radiotherapist to assure seamless integration of therapeutic suggestions. I now also search for and bring back newer therapies and practice them in the US, if FDA approved--and out of the US, if not FDA approved. Through my patients' generous financial support to the Biofoundation for Angiogenesis Research and Development, I am able to discover, evaluate and incorporate better treatment protocols into my practice.

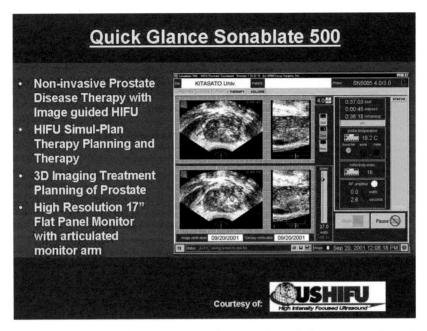

Fig. 5.1 2001 example of non invasive ultrasound guided treatment from Japan

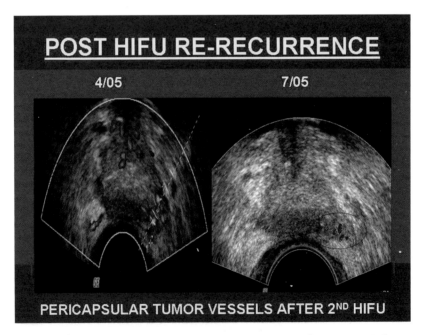

Fig.5.2 15% of aggressive tumors may recur or re-recur after sequential treatments

CHAPTER SIX

Options for Treating Prostate Cancer

Primum non nocere from the sacred physician's Hippocratic Oath, means "First, Do No Harm." This chapter is designed to give the reader a sense of what cancer is, how the newer treatments work and how to use this information in his personal life. Some readers are extremely knowledgeable about cancer and cancer treatments; and for other patients, this book is the very first information they have been able to read to find out more about cancer options. This time in the cancer patient's life is tremendously frightening as well as bewildering for him. In order for the book to be useful and valuable, I invite the reader to think about how the material presented could make a difference in addressing his particular personal health problems or perhaps, the health problems of a loved one.

The reader needs to study with an open mind about cancer and about what to expect from this book. A useful way to interact with this text is through the readers' search for new ideas; for example, how other people have fared in their cancer cure search, what methods friends have used successfully in dealing with cancer, what researchers and physicians worldwide have discovered and written, and then comparing this with what the cancer societies promote as "accepted" facts. If the reader involves himself this way, he still might only obtain more evidence to support his already formed opinions or he might become enlightened. It is human nature to want to be right; so subconsciously, one gathers evidence to support his preconceived ideas and turn opinions into facts. The reader can either keep his opinions or have access to possibilities. Gleaning value from the material presented requires an open mind and a thirst for knowledge to significantly make a difference in impacting prostate health.

There are ways of interpreting or evaluating information with which the reader may not be familiar. Some of these principles are reviewed in this book. When people read, they actually read through a filter. For example, if a person puts on a pair of yellow sunglasses, everything would appear yellow. However, if the person leaves them on for a week, things wouldn't appear yellow, they would appear "normal." This is called the "already-always way of reading." We have many other filters in our lives. Perhaps we relate to the filter as if our perceptions are real. Perhaps it's only an "already-always" way of thinking.

Take this question: What does everyone know about teen-agers? A man thinks, "That's the way my teenagers are." He simply accepts all preconceived ideas. A more powerful way of reading this book is for an individual not to filter the information in the text so that he can completely utilize it and make a significant difference in his life. A person should read and digest the information for his own personal and unique needs, but in a way that he may not ordinarily consider.

A personal example of the "already-always" thinking is the day my car was towed away. I had parked legally in front of my office on East 60th street in the early evening. When I stepped out, I saw a police tow truck towing my car down the block. I had apparently failed to see a small paper sign warning of a movie shooting sequence on the street and allowing no parking during that time period. At any rate, as I saw the Department of Transportation truck cross over Park Avenue with my vehicle dangling in the back, I knew that I would have to recover my car later from the tow pound by the Hudson River piers on the west side of town. I knew it would take a few hours to tag the car in the system before I could recover it. I called up at midnight, and the car was not in the pound. "Call back later," said the officer. By 2:00 A.M. the car had not yet been logged into the data base. I decided to wait until the next day. Many calls throughout the day netted me no information of the whereabouts of my car. I finally spoke with the desk sergeant and told him from where my car had been removed. He checked with the temporary towing department, and informed me that my car had been moved a block and a half west of my original parking spot. Worse, was the realization that I had walked past it several times that day in broad daylight and not recognized it; since, I "knew" it had be towed away to the pound on the west side.

A sadder example occurred with a family from New Jersey. My patient brought in his family for screening ever since I had found his aortic aneurysm (ballooning of the abdominal main artery) and saved his life. He understood the value of periodic ultrasound screening. One day he brought with him his niece, a healthy looking middle aged woman, who had a normal abdominal sonogram. When I continued the scan to her pelvis, I found a large tumor which was asymptomatic. It turned out she had a breast cancer treated nine years ago and had been in stable remission. She went to her oncologist with the results of my scan. He told her the tumor had spread, and there was nothing he could do other than palliative treatment to keep her comfortable. Two weeks later her abdomen filled with fluid from the tumor, and 10 days afterwards she passed away. The family thinks that the hopeless prognosis accelerated her early demise. She listened to her doctors' pronouncement and took it as a death sentence. She could have heard it as a wake-up call to empower her healing mechanisms. The types of people who get sick are ordinary, every-day people. They cover a full spectrum of age and characteristics. They vary from youngsters in their thirty's to men in their ninety's! Some are rich men and some are poor men! Some are famous and some are anonymous. Prostate cancer in the 21st century does not discriminate by age, fame or wealth.

My teaching techniques used in this book are not like traditional education, where one studies and learns. That kind of education is referred to as linear. What I try to do in the text is distinct from that in two ways: the first is in the issues addressed, and the second is in the approach. The issues I address are questions patients have in every day life, such as, how can I be more effective in treating my disease, how do I improve my diet, how do I pep-up my immune system, how do I have a sexually satisfying life, etc.

It could be said that health education is additive—where an individual studies and learns, and the more he puts in, the more he gets out. What is accomplished in the book is non-linear; in fact, the text is a systematic approach to non-linear learning. It can be paralleled in concept to the kind of work that scientists seek to achieve. When scientists work, (and I am a scientist), they dwell in a problem, dwell in an issue, or dwell in a specific area to find a breakthrough. They carefully examine all facets of the problem to find a reasonable solution. They have done all the preparation, obtained all the available information, and keep bumping up against questions and struggling against answers and brainstorming for solutions; then, there's an "all-of-a-sudden" phenomenon or epiphany that happens. It is very much like turning a light on in a dark room. When this phenomenon happens, they suddenly see something they have never seen before. It all comes together--something is made possible that was never possible before. Now, that's the kind of awakening I wish for the reader to experience from this book. A break through often occurs while dwelling in the areas that a person doesn't know he is blind or ignorant about.

Everyone actually has had a similar experience in his own life. For example, learning to ride a bicycle is like that. A man learns important skills directly connected to riding a bicycle; he practices, he fall off, he get back on the bike, and then "all of a sudden" he grasps what balance is, and the whole experience comes together like a completed puzzle. It's the same way with scientific discovery. Most people have had this kind of discovery experience; yet, they don't have direct access to its secret or the comprehension of how it all happened when it is discovered. It happens by accident, and everyone hopes that they will experience it again. In this book, the reader is actually given the tools to access that kind of experience in his search for a healthy life.

My approach to health involves a change in perspective. It is important to understand the working process of any complex entity, be it the interactive parts of an automobile or the inner dynamics of the human body. For example, take the automobile--if the only thing a man knows about the automobile is that there is a steering wheel to guide the car, gasoline to make it run, a radio to play, windows to look out and air conditioning to enjoy in hot weather, the lack of knowledge could be a disaster when a breakdown occurs. And, if he lifted the hood to look beneath it, what he would see is something "black and dirty." Now, another person who is knowledgeable about cars could lift up the same hood and see spark plugs, pistons, carburetors, etc. If you are stuck because your car won't start, which of the above persons would you want to work on it? The man who understands the working parts of an automobile has a better chance to solve the problem with someone who is a good mechanic. So too, is the man who understands the working parts of his own body more able to interact better with and extract more from his physician. For example, I know the prostate has benign enlargements that are being successfully treated by laser. I know lasers reduce bleeding by destroying blood vessels. I have brought the concept of using lasers to destroy vascular tumors to the attention of my urologic colleagues and we will start a joint study in the near future to treat small prostate cancers with a technology used to reduce benign disease.

Everyone has specific techniques or methods to use to obtain access to his medical problems. It isn't something that is impossible to control or that is locked up and can only be accessed by doctors. Most of the medical problems involve how a person lives, how he thinks, and what he perceives as health possibilities, etc. Cancer has its own set of working principles. To have access to this is to have power regarding disease and control over one's health. One specific tool underused is listening to your doctor. Men don't want to hear bad news, yet that is the access to power. Negative findings are like a red flag. It is necessary information to take charge of a problem. Verify with your physician what you heard by repeating it back and asking for a written report. I speak with my patients initially, then hand them a written report and ask them to read it and speak with me again. If you are unclear, call back the same day or as soon as possible to have your questions answered. Remember that there are no stupid questions. This is your health! No, this is your life at stake! Do not ask for certainty, but get clarity about available options and side effects.

Let me give you personal examples of "incomplete" listening. The German's have a popular phrase for this kind of discontinuous communication: *Sie reden einander vorbei,* translated, meaning: "they speak past one another". I believe in aerobic exercise for health and I take weekly ballroom dancing lessons. There is a big sign in the dance studio that reads: I KNOW YOU HEARD WHAT I SAID, BUT WHAT YOU THINK I TOLD YOU IS NOT WHAT I MEANT YOU TO DO. There is a standard dance step called the cross body lead. The man steps back and guides his partner past him across his body. The mans body moves 90 degrees away from the woman thus opening a door like a swinging gate allowing the woman to dance straight ahead through the opening he has just created. 99% of men, including myself who has been taking dance lessons for over twenty years, do not open the door for the woman like a hinged gate but, rather, step away at an angle. I did this and told my instructor I had followed the directions to the letter. When the video was replayed, I was astounded that my mind told me my body was acting according to the given instructions even though my body was moving in a direction different from my strict intentions. My dance instructor now judges the effectiveness of communication by what people do rather than what they say they understand.

This analogy is applicable to my patients, since I follow up and verify what happens clinically at a 3 to 6 months interval. Most failures stem from non compliance of therapeutic instructions-specifically, some men stop treatment when they feel better, some stop to try other regimens, some substitute impure foreign made antioxidants for American made products, some reduce the effectiveness by taking other pills and herbs that neutralize the treatment regimen, etc.

A variation of incomplete listening is "negative listening" Being human means making assumptions. Assumptions make an ass out of your subject and make an ass out of the assumer. Fifteen years ago I attended a state wide conference of radiologists specializing in mammography and breast imaging at NYU Medical Center. My associate, Dr. Strax, had been using a high intensity light device to transilluminate the breast for cancer for 30 years with remarkable success. He had trained me in this technique and I found it clinically useful as an adjunct to the breast sonography I performed. At this conference, a question was asked from the keynote speaker: *"Is any one in the audience working with breast transillumination?"* As I was raising my hand in a room filled with 250 specialists, I found that my arm was the only one visible in a sea of unimpressed faces. Nevertheless, I kept my hand up as my self esteem fell. Two months later I received a call from the pathology department at NYU Medical Center. The Director of Pathology introduced himself and I braced myself for the worst. Did I misdiagnose a breast cancer? Is the patient all right? The chief pathologist was also an editor of a major cancer journal and had received a paper from the Republic of China on their positive experience with breast transillumination as a diagnostic modality. Before he would accept the article for publication, he asked the NYU Radiology Department what they knew about this technique. No one had any idea, but a staff member remembered my courage in admitting my use of a newer technology, and provided my number to the journal reviewer. As I affirmed the validity of the technique, my relief was only equaled by my pride as an innovator. Eight years ago, early on in my diagnostic prostate work I was referred a VIP from a highly esteemed university hospital physician. The gentleman had an erratic PSA history and no family history of prostate cancer. He had no mass on the rectal exam or urinary symptoms. The sonogram showed a large vascular aggressive tumor. He went back, visibly shaken, to his primary care physician. A week later I get a fax from the referring doctor that the patient was biospied and *"everything is fine."* I became doubtful about the accuracy of my work and started getting depressed. A few days following, I ran into the primary doctor who congratulated me on my finding which forced the VIP to have a biopsy and discover a significant tumor. The phrase *"everything is fine."* meant that the cancer was removed before it had spread. It is a useful practice to assign no particular meaning to words. It is better to check out the intention directly from the originator of the communication both for clarity of message and for stability of blood pressure.

In May 2005 there was an assemblage of physicians and scientists from all over the world to report their studies of a new technique to shrink the prostate. There were urologists, pharmacists, internists and radiologists present at this meeting in San Antonio, Texas discussing new injection techniques. Every one was in general agreement until the urologists said they injected their drug into the sides of the enlarged prostate. The radiologists jumped up and cried out that the middle of the prostate enlarges and not the sides. The urologists shouted back that they always did their surgery on the lateral lobes not the middle lobe. The radiologists showed pictures that the middle or central zone is the enlarged area. After a few minutes of heated debate, it became obvious that both parties were correct. We had been looking at an elephant from different vantage points. The MRI and sonogram show the enlarged central zone of the prostate correctly. The urologist looks at the prostate from the urethra in the middle of the prostate so the enlargement appears to be coming from both lateral sides. The commitment to improve this new treatment was stronger than the desire to be right about their valid opinions. By giving up the "truth," each group developed a better understanding of a highly complex problem. In 2006, the NIH gave a grant to a New York hospital to evaluate botox injections to shrink the prostate. This was the same hospital that had earlier dismissed the process as potentially dangerous several years earlier.

SHIFTING THE LIMITS OR PARADIGMS IN WHICH A PERSON OPERATES

What is a paradigm? Essentially a paradigm defines the limits of the way each person perceives life around him or the way he defines his world. It's a pattern or mold that each man follows. It is a precise learned way of thinking. It might be perceived that I am talking about "culture"; it is sort of a background phenomenon—a way of thinking or knowing something. An American, for example, has certain ways of perceiving his "Americanism" that are obvious, but when he goes to another culture, people think very differently about those same things because of their backgrounds—or the paradigms or the basic invisible limits that mold their thinking from which they develop their ideas and/or perceptions are very different.

For example, when I was lecturing at the Mayo Clinic division in Scottsdale, Arizona in 1994, I had occasion to be in a fabric store in nearby Phoenix, Arizona. I saw a pretty umbrella in a stand by the door. When I asked how much it was, they said: "It's not for sale. We're in the desert. Here umbrellas are used only for decoration." If the salesperson could have shifted the idea that umbrellas are not only for rain, he could have advertised and sold them for protection from the sun. This would have been utilizing possibilities by thinking outside the box.

One can say that in shifting away from old ideas and assumptions, from where a person normally begins his thought processes, he can create whole new possibilities for moving his life forward and actually breaking through to accept new, dynamic ideas. It's not merely that he going to try out a different solution, it's that "what is" in the foreground entirely changes.

Here are several examples: Centuries ago, people used to think evil spirits caused disease, and the methods of curing disease ranged from drilling holes in heads to let out the evil spirits, to "bleeding" patients. Next, germs and bacteria were discovered. That discovery completely altered the entire field of medicine and the possibilities of how to diagnose and treat disease.

Another way to exemplify what I mean by operating outside the current paradigm is exemplified by the 9 dots puzzle below. Thinking outside the box is a valuable way to stretch the imagination. The object in solving this game is to connect all 9 dots without removing the pencil from the paper and using a continuous and uninterrupted line.

9 DOTS PUZZLE

To solve the puzzle, one must connect all 9 dots by using four straight connected lines. The lines must be continuous. Most everyone tries to solve this inside the box because that's the normal paradigm in which most people think. But, when one goes outside of the box, whole new solutions are possible. Simply extending line 1 past the last dot opens up a previously unpredictable possibility.

9 DOTS PUZZLE SOLVED

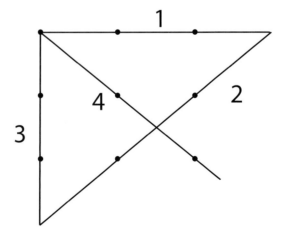

In 1968 Switzerland had dominated the world of watch making for the previous 60 years. The Swiss made the best watches in the world. Anyone who wanted a good, accurate time piece bought a Swiss watch. They were the leaders in watch making by an enormous stretch. Yet, by 1980 their market share had collapsed from 65 percent where it was in 1968 to less than 10 percent. By all significant measures, they had been dethroned as the world market leader in making watches. What happened?

They had run into a paradigm shift—a change in the fundamental rules of watch making. This was a different way of doing something. The mechanical mechanism was about to give way to electronics. Everything the Swiss were good at became irrelevant with the advent of advanced electronics. The Swiss themselves had invented the electronic quartz movement. Yet, when the Swiss researchers presented this revolutionary new idea to the Swiss manufacturers in 1967, it was rejected. After all, it didn't have a mainspring, it didn't need bearings, it required almost no gears, and, because it was electronic, it was powered by batteries instead of by winding. It couldn't possibly be the watch of the future. For another nation, however, it was the opportunity of a lifetime. Seiko took one look and the rest is history. They comprehended the possibilities of cordless clocks and watches that never needed to be wound. Another powerful example is: 600 years ago every body knew the world was flat. It was the only paradigm available at the time, and everyone operated consistent with this idea, such as not sailing over the horizon. When it was discovered that the world was round, whole new possibilities become available.

A classic example of science overruled by bureaucracy occurred when a young Hungarian physician, named Ignaz Semmelweis, discovered that a contagious disease was being transmitted to hospital patients because the treating personnel failed to wash their hands. In the 1800's, tens of thousands of women died every year due to puerperal sepsis (childbirth fever). The cause for this epidemic was that doctors were performing autopsies and then conducting vaginal pelvic examinations with their hands still covered with decomposing tissue of the dead subjects. Dr. Semmelweis made the observation that women delivered by midwives instead of doctors had lower rates of the deadly childbirth fever. Semmelweis, in an experiment to prove his assumption that the postpartum infection was due to contamination spread by cadaver to the womb, required his staff to wash their hands with disinfectant prior to attending patients. The mortality rate dropped from 18% to 1%. Upon publication of his findings, the medical community reacted with hostility, since the belief in the 19th century was that "bad air" caused the fever. Tragically, due his unfaltering attempts to persuade his skeptical colleagues, Semmelweis was committed to an insane asylum where he died at the age of forty two years.

When fleas are placed in a jar with a lid cover, the fleas will jump until they hit the lid. After the lid is removed they still only jump as high as the lid. That limit became the extent of their paradigm even though, in actuality, far more room to jump was available. Human beings, including physicians, are sometimes similar to fleas. For example, when some people express themselves too freely, they get hurt. If this happens repetitively, they withdraw to protect themselves. Because they are vulnerable to pain, they give themselves invisible limits. Unfortunately, people live in safe and comfortable mindsets where life is limited but "bearable." Physicians, too, are afraid to try new treatments and are understandably satisfied with their current routines. Patients may consider jumping out of the jar when their current options do not look promising.

An allied state is being alert to opportunities that are unexpected. The chairman of a world wide Japanese electronic company had a daughter who was born mentally defective with Down's syndrome. Although he loved his child, he was greatly distressed at the high odds of having another disabled infant. Since he was a music aficionado and believed in the healing power of this medium, he devised a sound system to play music inside the womb of his newly pregnant wife. These external speakers would be attached to the abdomen and project the sound waves into the uterus so the maturing fetus would be bathed in pleasant vibrations while floating in its fluid compartment. Soon thereafter a manufacturing error produced a massive supply of radios without speakers. Unphased, he attached his headphones to external output of the speakerless product and invented, yes, the *walkman!* Taking action raises our antennae to new possibilities. You may create history also.

The book provides the ability to identify the paradigms from which the reader is thinking. A person might not even be cognizant of the trap or limited situation his mind is in. It gives the reader access to invent new paradigms for himself that give him a far broader range of possibilities. He may want to ask himself: What are the imaginary boxes I'm living confined in? What treatments are available that I'm not even aware of? If I wait, will there be new and better therapies next year? When the patient makes this connection of new possibilities, he regains "hope." He is able to see light at the end of the tunnel. He perceives something that he hasn't been able to perceive before. He realizes a wide variety of therapies that treat cancer and manage disease are now available to choose at his doorstep. Please read of the inspirational health crusade undertaken by one of my Australian patients in his e-mail to a prostate cancer alternative group displayed as follows:

2005 e-mail letter from AUSTRALIA:

i was dxd with pc in 1996 at age 45 and was almost bullied into a RP..however i told the urologist (one of the top ones in sydney at st vincents hospital) that he had no idea what he was doing to all these young men and i proceeded to give him the statistics...(over 70% recurrence within 8 years following a RP...in the years to come he actually told me that he would never have one himself!!!)....

i was fortunate to have the resources to abandon my business life for a time and travel the world looking for a cure...my path led me to bejing, china (i was chairman of a company building thousands of houses for the government) where i was "inspected" by the head of the cancer hospital and then by deng's personal physician, and then another expert who travelled 30 hours from mongolia..they all said the same thing...my body was out of balance with too much "yang"...the chinese believe that the body can only be in a state of "disease" if the yin/yang balance is disturbed and this in turn causes a blockage of "chi" or energy, prana, electrical current or whatever you call it...they also believe that the body has yin and yang organs...the yin organs being the "wet" ones ,liver, kidneys, pancreas, digestive system and the yang organs,"dry" and the heart, brain and lungs...the yin organs are the ones that control and monitor the immune system and cancer is an autoimmune disease so the key is to fix the immune system.

yang organs are boosted by adrenaline (fight or flight syndrome which inflicts the western world and is part of our way of life, constantly dribbling the dreaded chemicals whenever the phone rings) and the yin organs are boosted by balance and harmony (meditation, prayer, quiet etc)...it all made sense to me so after 3 weeks a treatment by a chi master i returned home feeling amazing.

i cleaned out my body with a 10 day fast, and a colema regime based on bernard jensen's philosophy, took up meditation again (i was a TM meditator 20 years earlier so was easy to fall right back in) and consumed vast amounts of stinking chinese herbs that i had brought home...my psa started to fall.

i read a lot of books by deepak chopra and his mind/body connection made a lot of sense...i had been a property developer for 20 years with lots of staff, debt and with an A type personality that was constantly pushing life's boundaries...(its interesting to note that PC is a disease of mostly A type personalities...there is 2.5 times the amount of PC in the US congress than the general population...all A types, bad diet, travel and constant fight or flight syndrome.) so i thought deepak was my man...i took a plane to san diego to meet and greet him...we became friends and i travelled to india with him constantly absorbing his healing message which is deeply reflective of the chinese, indian philosophy based around the mind/ body relationship and life balance, meditation etc...one of the first things deepak said to me was "andrew, what is causing this dis—ease ...look at your life and tell me"...i knew so very soon after this i got a divorce and set out with a new partner...my marriage was toxic and i knew deep down that it was making me ill.

around this stage i became aware of larry clapp and was amazed how close his philosophy and healing path was to the one i had developed for myself.... i also became aware of sophie chen and pc-spes so i jumped on that chat group and for 5 years took her concoction...the results of all this was great with my psa normal at about 2, my life rearranged and i was meeting a great bunch of guys through the site.... of course all this went when the discovery was made that tiny amounts of prescription drugs (DES) was in the purported herbal capsules and greedy men started to sue and reported the company, botaniclabs, to the authorities.... thus one of the best PC mixtures was banned and to this date no one has been able to replicate the formula...although Dr DONBACH is having success with his similar formula.

I have an annual checkup with my very clever friend, dr robert bard in new york and in february he declared me cancer free although my last psa test was about 6.... he says to ignore this and stop having it done.

i am fit and well and have sired another child recently (i now have 4), i am back building a few buildings but gently and without the extreme passion of days gone...i ran into the urologist (who wanted to operate in 1996 and told me i would be dead in three years if i didnt pay heed) at a party last xmas...he said he was still doing biopsies and RPs but really didn't believe they worked (what a dangerous path this guy is travelling...and i read in a sydney paper that he had bought a $6 million dollar house, so business must be good at $10,000 a pop) and he was now asking his patients to make up their own minds about the type of treatment path they chose rather than trying to bully them as he had done me.

so guys even though none of us asked to join this club we are all in it and helping each other...i believe my diagnosis has been a great gift in that it has lead me to all sorts of changes and new friends and situations...my "gods" have so far been very kind.

love and good health.
andrew richardson

Andrew J Richardson
Sydney

The following is a personal example of how this ability to shift paradigms has worked for me. My office building, a professional co-op, was constructed in 1920 at

121 East 60th Street off of Park Avenue. One day the panel door of the main fuse box opened up and couldn't be closed. The superintendent tried to force it, to push it, to jam it and to re adjust the frame to no avail. "Since these doors are no longer made, we will have to ask a machinist to make one similar to fit the opening," he said. Horrified at the thought of welders and electricians working in the corridor, I rethought the problem. What really bothered me was the fact that the ajar piece of metal looked out of place. As soon as the thought "ugly" popped into my head, I went into the waiting room, grabbed a painting off the wall and put it over the uncooperative opening. By re-focusing on what really was important, I was able to resolve the issue. Similarly, I had a bump under the wall-to-wall carpeting in my office. I called up the contractor and asked him to bring his flooring specialist to pull up the carpet and remove the offending object. He came over, looked at the protrusion in the middle of the fabric, took out his hammer and smashed the area flat. Another problem solved by alternative thinking.

Another personal experience occurred when I was at the gym on Lexington Avenue. I had just finished my workout when I heard the boiler had broken rendering no hot water available for the showers. I thought that by waiting the water problem would pass. It didn't. I decided to wait again and take a long session in the steam room. After fifteen minutes, I was ready for a bath, but the plumbing was not yet fixed. Once I realized that the pipes in the sauna and steam room area were hot, I went to the shower fixture, stood directly underneath, pulled the metal chain and got a five second deluge of warm water. Possibilities are made, not found.

As I was writing this chapter, a physician in our professional complex came in for an x-ray of his nose. He had injured his nose during a tennis match that morning. After I read the x-rays that suggested a fracture rather than confirmed one, I asked myself if there was a better way to look at the tiny bones in the nasal area. I had just read an article about x-rays missing 90 percent of rib fractures. X-rays of curved bones do not see all the borders. I knew from performing sonograms of the rotator cuff in the shoulder that I could detect fractures of the humerus better than the routine x-rays. I had also diagnosed wrist dislocations and rib fractures with regular sonogram techniques for years. However, as Chief of Radiology in 1980 at Manhattan's Eye and Ear Hospital, I knew how difficult fractures of the nose were to diagnose—even with dedicated x-ray equipment.

I wondered if I could perform a 3-D scan on the injured area. The 3-D probe for the "small parts" of the body is 4 cm or 2 inches wide and is usually used for breast or thyroid imaging. I thought of mustard on a hot dog in a bun. My idea was to let the hot dog be the nose and allow the bun be a container that holds a large quantity of ultrasound "gel" or coupling agent (mustard, in the analogy) in which the large probe face could rest. Then, I placed surgical tape to make receptacle for the gel around the nose sparing the nostrils, filled the area to the top with coupling material and obtained a beautiful 3-D picture of the nasal bones showing definite but non-displaced fractures on both sides.

Another method or "working principle" I use is called "paradox resolution." The French have a way they refer to what we're talking about in an adage they use: "Plus que ca change. Plus que ca reste le meme" "The more things change, the more they remain the same." That's paradoxical; and yet, it represents the nature of man's relationship to change. For example, I went to the ophthalmology department at New York Hospital to look at a new ultra high resolution ultrasound machine. This was being used to find defects in the cornea (surface of the eye) and I was hoping to use it in detecting skin cancers. When I asked the director of research about his experience with malignant melanoma, a highly vascular, extremely lethal skin malignancy, he looked surprised and told me that Doppler flow studies were not done in the eye. The American College of Ophthalmology, many years ago, concluded that there may be adverse side effects from this diagnostic procedure. No dedicated eye scanners in the United States are using the Doppler technology today. When I mentioned that the Europeans were using this to diagnose the aggressiveness of eye tumors, great interest was generated. Suddenly, I had ophthalmologists trying my equipment on their own eyes to observe the normal blood flow to the retina (back of eye). Dr. Robert Ritch, surgeon director of New York Eye and Ear Infirmary, and I are evaluating the use of this technology in diagnosing the severity of glaucoma (increase eye pressure causing blindness). We have shown that the greater the pressure inside the eyeball, the lower the amount of blood to enter. This now provides a diagnostic tool and a potential measure of the effectiveness of treatment since the blood flow increases as the successful therapy decreases the eye pressure. One never knows what will become possible when paradigms shift. New opportunities often arise. Consider the following anonymous quote: "The conversation you have with yourself after you dive off the high diving board is quite different from the one you had while you were climbing up the ladder."

Human beings are designed to resist or change things that are unwanted, unpleasant or irritating to them. That's just the way our human "machinery" works—so to speak. When the reader comprehends the actual "design mechanism" in cancer, he will have a new power over the outcome and be able to control the results and better endure the process. How many people have been trying to change events in their lives? For example, people try to change their relationship with children, or projects at work, or diets, or some quality involving them. How many people try to change the same things for a long period of time without success? What's paradoxical is that a man's zsolution as disappearing vs. changing, which provides an alternative to changing the issues with which man struggles. It gives him a powerful way to relate to these problems, so that they actually clear up or disappear as significant issues. You can't change the fact that you have cancer and complaining certainly will not make any difference. You can, however, make promises and requests. Promises such as: I will drink green tea and alter my diet, I will engage in aerobic exercises, I will search the internet for new treatments, etc. Requests such as: I will ask men about successful treatments, I will find support groups, I will tell my family and friends to assist me in lifestyle changes, I will contribute to cancer foundations, etc.

An example that is common in my practice is erectile dysfunction, (ED). The very thought of a prostate problem robs men of libido. The threat of prostate surgery produces fear and stress which often leads to impotence. While this can't be changed, the option of non-invasive therapies or minimally invasive treatments improves men's sexual performance. Additionally, drugs such as Cialis and Viagra permit satisfactory sex lives when undergoing the various hormone castration protocols. The new and effective health alternatives render current problems less frustrating. A more graphic expression would be the following: imagine a bad mosquito bite on the arm torturing a man, now imagine if the man's other arm were cut off with a chain saw, then the merciless itching will no longer be bothersome because his focus has changed. A powerful commitment is the best antidote to being obsessive about one's worries.

CREATING A TEAM

Teamwork forwards events more effectively and frequently faster. I consider my patients as part of my team. Men and often, their wives, forward successful outcomes to my attention as well as negative treatment side effects. For example, women with breast cancer have reported control of their tumor by injections of *botulinum neuro-toxin a or b* (Botox or Myobloc) in and around the abnormal growth. No side effects have been described from this. One of my patient's heard about this and decided to try this on his recurrent prostate cancer. He had radiation for Gleason 9 disease and had a recurrence 10 months later. This was treated with HIFU but the tumor recurred again. In despair, his recurrence was injected with neurotoxin in Europe resulting in stabilization for six months. At his half year follow up, the treated area was inactive but a new tumor occurred on the opposite side. He had repeat HIFU therapy and both sides are stable at his 1 year follow up.

One reason to build a health care team is to reduce human error. Errors result from the natural physiological and psychological limitations of human beings. Sources of error are commonly: fatigue, workload, mental overload, poor interpersonal communications, imperfect information processing and flawed decision making. Imagine a staircase: at the bottom is a step called *fatigue*. The next level may be called *team creation*. A step above this is designated *recognition of adverse situations*. On top of this is *communications*. The pinnacle level is *decision making*.

Managing fatigue occurs when we are rested and properly nutritioned. Yoga and exercise are both stress reducers leading to higher mental functioning and stronger physical status. Team creation is necessary since no one person can do it all in today's complex world. Each team member must have an area of personal responsibility. For example, the physician provides treatment, the patient follows a planned therapy, the wife or nurse makes sure the patient keeps his commitment to health, family members offer support, etc. The more members in a team, the greater the chance of catching and correcting any errors. On a practical note, the presence of an effective team enhances communication and reduces stress through overall better performance.

Effective use of a team requires an invitation to participate in your care. One must encourage team members to provide information, express their concerns and speak up when necessary. The patient must show respect for all the team and put his ego below the good intentions of the support group. Imaging saying, "Botox is for women" and turning off any future possibility that may derive from an open mind. The industrialist, Henry Ford put teamwork this way "Coming together is a beginning. Keeping together is progress. Working together is success."

An important function of the team is to recognize adverse situations by looking for red flags or warning signs. The usual indicators of adversity are: conflicting information, preoccupation, poor communication and departure from usual practice. At the first sign of adversity, others must be sought out actively. Let us say the physician has had a rough day and is both stressed and fatigued. He may be curt or distracted or both. You may hear: "This is an aggressive tumor" at the beginning of the visit and "Let me see you in six months" and the end of the consultation. Signs of poor doctor communication include talking too much and/or not listening to you. Signs of poor patient communication include stressing unimportant test results (such as PSA) and thinking you understand fully what is being said. This includes not addressing discrepancies such as becoming anemic at the same time the PSA drops. As the patient, you have the right to demand specific measurable performance from each member of your health team. Remember, the design of the team is to assist you in making the best health care decisions possible. So keep your team well oiled and you will have a smoother ride through your illness. Perhaps your support group is negative and continually warns you that every cancer is deadly and the treatments are worse than dying. If you can't empower them with a presentation of up to date facts, take action and change support groups. It is your responsibility to make your life better. You must realize that there are no victimizers, only willing victims. Your health in ultimately in your hands and your doctor is part of your health team. Men who take charge of their lives more often prevail against prostate cancer.

A mission for a team to develop new treatments might look like this: Ask a PC survivor to grow a designated herb in a garden, take it for half a year and report what happens to an assigned person. Then ask him to request two other men to do the same with different plants and have each of the two new participants to enroll another two men to follow suit. It has been estimated 25% of the plant botanical varieties have been identified to date. Countless potential herbal sources are available to be studied. This scenario could create a team of 100,000 men and hundreds of new medical treatments within one year. How would you like to multiply your chances for beating cancer and living a fuller life? The hardest part of progress is to take a first step. Make it a small one, if you must, but start immediately. If it doesn't work out, start again. Action takes the sting out of defeat, buffers the misery of disease and moves us forward out of despair.

I always recall the Hippocratic oath: **First do no harm. Primum non nocere.** What are the likely side effects of standard diagnostic tests and treatment formats? It is important to observe the procedure for the commonplace prostate biopsy. A patient must be off blood thinners for at least a week and off Plavix for two weeks. Antibiotics must be taken before and after the biopsies for three days. The routine sextant (6 core) biopsy often misses the front or anterior part of the gland where 24 percent of cancers may arise and may miss centrally located tumors in the back or posterior part of the gland. Spread of bacteria into the blood occur, which may affect diseased heart valves or other weakened organs. Life threatening complications of severe bleeding and major infection occur in 1 percent of patients. Spread of the tumor into the biopsy tract is common, although the significance of this is not fully established. Mild complications such as blood in the urine and sperm are reported at 24 percent and 45 percent respectively. Low grade fever occurs in 5 percent. Painful voiding or difficult urination occurs in 13 percent. Dr. C. Naughton, in the 1998 report in the journal *Urology* noted that the standard sextant, 3 passes right lobe and 3 passes left lobe, biopsy protocol will miss 64 percent of cancers in larger glands. "Large" is defined as volume over 60 cc (three times larger than the normal 20 cc). To remedy this situation, urologists are now performing "saturation" biopsies, ranging from 24 to 96 samples. When one considers the volume of prostate sampled this way, only about 1–2% of the prostate mass is actually removed for pathologic analysis according to a presentation at the 2007 AUA meeting by Dr. George Suarez.

One of my medical colleagues had a routine biopsy for rising PSA and happily no cancer was found. However, his prostate became infected and he was admitted to the hospital. The antibiotics were not successful and the infection spread to his bladder. A new antibiotic still did not suppress the inflammation and it spread to his bone. Nine months later, significant because he was an obstetrician, he was delivered from the hospital after an experimental drug managed to control the infectious process. He lost his practice and is still only capable of working part time. He had to undergo extensive drug rehabilitation since he became addicted to the narcotics necessary to reduce his pain.

Little discussed in the literature is the possibility that the needle biopsy may itself initiate the spread of prostate cancer. In the cause of a cancer confined within the prostate capsule, introduction of the biopsy needle may facilitate spread beyond the capsule into the seminal vesicles or peri-rectal space. The medical term for disease caused by the medical staff is "iatrogenic" This phenomenon of tumor spread is termed, variously, as "iatrogenic seeding," "needletrack seeding" or "iatrogenic metastasis" Dr. The, in the2001 *Journal of Urology,* noted the dissemination of cancer following radioactive seed therapy and surgical resections.

Dr. H. Hricak, Director of Radiology for Memorial Hospital gave a presentation (full text is in appendix at end of book) in 2005 at New York Roentgen Society Meeting which reviewed statistics from Memorial Sloan Kettering Cancer Center highlighting the fact routine biopsies missed about 80 percent of all cancers, and the pathologic results from interpretation of these biopsies is accurate in 58 percent of readings as compared with the final pathology report from the surgically removed prostate. It was suggested that biopsies be performed based on imaging findings of MRI. Drs. Robert Grubb and Peter Choyke, physicians from the National Institute of Health, presented a 2005 paper at the American Urological Association Meeting with their experience in biopsies of the prostate using a MRI guided transrectal prostate biopsy protocol. Their conclusion was that this is a safe and accurate procedure that will improve the lack of specificity of the PSA test and find cancers where the biopsy has previously missed. Indeed, Dr. Barentsz, President of the International Cancer Imaging Society, noted that one patient had 55 biopsies miss the cancer before the MRI guided procedure found the mass. When I gave a lecture to a prostate cancer survivor's group at Hackensack Medical Center in New Jersey in 2006, one of the men raised his hand and stated that he had undergone 86 biopsies before his cancer was discovered. He had never shared that before because he was ashamed that he was so unusually difficult for the biopsy to be successful.

In my own four year series of 899 patients studied with 3D PDS ultrasound and MRI scans taken within a week, the findings revealed a 95 percent correlation between the ultrasound and the DCE-MRI results. Indeed, a recent patient had a normal biopsy and a rising PSA. When I scanned his prostate, I saw a large tumor in the center of the gland just out of the range of the usual biopsy sites of the classic sextant biopsy. Many patients who have had one or more biopsies refuse to have any more. Most feel it is better to deal with the possibility of cancer growing slowly than the certainty of the unpleasant side effects of the biopsy procedure. Another mant who had a successful robot radical prostatectomy one year earlier came in to evaluate a PSA that had risen from 0.2 to 0.8 ng/ml. His surgeon advised hormone therapy to stop the recurrence. His 3D-PDS was unremarkable for new tumor but disclosed a polyp in the bladder which was irregular and vascular. T DCE-MRI showed a normal postoperative prostate site and confirmed the bladder cancer. The patient was not only spared the unnecessary hormone shots, but probably had his life saved by the fortuitous discovery of a bladder malignancy which was becoming invasive.

A January 2005 review from the respected cancer information publication *Moss Reports* highlighted data from the June, 2004 Medical Forum of the John Wayne Cancer Institute in California. This Institute, through its St John's Hospital division, previously pioneered a procedure known as the sentinel node biopsy for staging spread of breast cancer to the glands. If the gland near the neck was involved, no further exploration of the nodes would be undertaken. Dr. Hansen's summarization of findings in 663 women who had breast cancer, half of whom had a biopsy with a needle prior to definitive surgery, showed that the probing by a metallic needle did increase the spread of the tumor to the glands by 50 percent. The breast biopsy is usually 2 to 4 biopsy extractions rather than the 6 to 18 currently in practice for prostate diagnosis. Extrapolation of this possible increased risk of cancer spread in men is not established as of this writing.

The side effects of the standard BPH treatment, the trans-urethral resection of the prostate, (TURP) are failures in 25 percent, death within 30 days at 0.4 percent for men 65–69 years and 2 percent for men 80–84 years. Twelve percent had immediate surgical complications. Two percent required repeat surgery from bleeding. There was erectile dysfunction in 14 percent and incontinence in 5 percent. Seventy-four percent had retrograde ejaculation. (sperm containing fluid goes backwards into the bladder instead of forward out the penis). A study by Drs. Alexis Te and J. S. Sandhu presented at the 100th American Urological Association Meeting in 2005 showed that the complication rate of TURP's is increasing. They feel it is due to the fact that residents in training are performing fewer procedures and warn that, if the trend continues, "TURP is not going to be a safe and readily available procedure in the near future." Fortunately, the green light laser procedure is becoming a better alternative to this procedure.

What causes or promotes prostate cancers? While there is no definitive agreement on the prime cause of prostate malignancy, there is a popularly held concept that it is promoted by excess testosterone. One might doubt this theory, since this cancer never strikes teenage boys or young men, who have peak testosterone levels at that age. It appears that a metabolite (breakdown products by the body's chemistry) of testosterone, dihydro-testosterone (DHT), is better linked to this disease. In later life, a greater amount of testosterone is converted to DHT. This is then converted into estrogen, which seems to be a potent stimulator of abnormal cell growth. The male hormone (androgen) comes from the testicles and the adrenal glands on top of each kidney. Current thinking suggests this hormone may aggravate prostate tumors.

Another, more recent and less accepted view, is the role of two steroids in the development of tumor aggression and was authored by Dr. W. Reid Pitts in the 2007 *British Journal of Urology.* For simplicity, the steroids are 5 AR (5-alpha-reductase) which converts testosterone to DHT and aromatase which converts testosterone to estradiol, a female estrogen type hormone. The theory is higher grade prostate cancers, Gleason Sums 8–10, are the product of low 5AR and increased aromatase. This evidence is gleaned from the large finasteride trial (Prostate Cancer Prevention Trial) and smaller trials on dutasteride. DHT contributes to cellular death of tumors. Estradiol binds to the androgen and estrogen receptors and mediates cellular proliferation. Finasteride and dutasteride inhibit 5-AR. Decreasing 5AR by 90% results in a 35 fold decrease in DHT, a 20 times increase in testosterone and a 19 fold increase in estrogen. In summary, low 5 AR results in unchecked prostatic cell proliferation due to increased estrogen unopposed by DHT.

More evidence is gained from the fact that dietary fat decreases the activity of 5 AR and the conversion of testerone to DHT. Japanese men have lower levels of 5 AR and DHT due to genetic differences from westerners. Although the prevalence of incidental prostate cancer is the same in Japanese men and American men, the death rate is much lower in Japan. First generation Japanese men in the US with a high fat western diet had an increase in prostate cancer deaths from 1.7/100,000 to 12.9/100,000 or 750 % jump in mortality. The fatty tissue in obese patients contains aromatase that produces high estrogen levels and accounts for increased risk of prostate cancer metastases. Aromatase inhibitors, commonly used for breast cancer patients, may be used as a chemoprevention for prostate cancer. Dr. Pitts likened the steroid pair to automotive functions, 5 AR is the *brake* on cancer and aromatase is the *accelerator* for tumor growth.

Hormone therapy consists of drugs and supplements counteracting the male hormone testosterone which promotes aggression in prostate cancers. Many treatments are successful, but one cannot tell which will work for a specific patient other than monitoring the PSA and symptoms. Drs. Lee and Bahn advocate treatment with Lupron and Zolodex to block the testicular hormones and Flutamide or Casodex to inhibit adrenal gland hormone secretion. Work with investigators from international centers has shown that effective hormone blockade will diminish the blood supply to the prostate in 1–7 weeks, as demonstrated by the 3-D PDS testing. Diminished libido, hot flashes, diarrhea, insomnia, liver damage and cardiovascular problems, tender and enlarging breasts are some of the side effects. A five year study by Dr. Shahinian published in the 2005 *New England Journal of Medicine* showed that the risk of fractures in men on hormone therapy is increased by 7 percent over the expected rate. Lately, this treatment has been used to shrink the tumor and the prostate volume so that other definitive therapies may be instituted. It is generally medically thought that this is a temporary measure for tumor control and the cancer will become refractory to the treatment in 3–5 years rendering the hormones no longer effective. This idea does not take into consideration the possibility of new or "interval cancers." Indeed, many of my long term hormone treatment survivors start taking hormonal substitutes when their PSA goes up or I find tumor re-growths. These treatments are generally helpful. One of my patients who returned every June for the past seven years shares this story:

This is his recent e-mail:

Edward Brenner

DOB 10/30/26 DX 5/98 PSA 4.8 Gleason 3+4 Aneuoploid

I have had no conventional treatment. For 24 months of the first 30 months I took PC Spes.

3/01 I began taking PC Plus which I am currently (6/05) taking. My PSA has ranged from as low as .1 to 4.5 which is its current level. PSA changes have been irregular probably effected by changes in PC Plus dosage.

I also take, and have been taking for a long time, many other supplements. The list pertaining to PCa includes lycopene, lutein, selenium, mixed E tocopherols, dry E succinate, Vitamin D-3, phytosterols, resveratrol, tocotrienols, curcumin, pumpkin seed oil, indole 3 carbinol, green tea, broccoli sprout powder, cod liver oil, calcium D-Glucarate, zinc, quercetin and ground flax seed. I take other supplements for general health.

I eat little red meat, dairy, or wheat, I exercise very moderately but fairly regularly.

I have had 7 power/color Doppler ultrasound exams each June by Dr. R. Bard in NYC and I have a semi-annual urological DRE exam. Dr. Bard's '04 exam showed no focal mass but his '05 exam has shown 2 significant tumors which were confirmed by MRI.

6/17/05

Radical Prostatectomy includes the surgical removal of the prostate and seminal vesicles.

Complications of radical prostatectomy for cancer, a major surgical procedure, are: incontinence–23 percent, impotence–85 percent and urinary obstruction–15 percent. Recovery is 2–3 weeks after 3 days in hospital. Cancer may reoccur in 20 percent. However, the Prostate Institute of America data shows that 55 percent of cancers thought to be localized to the prostate had actually escaped out of the prostate capsule. According to Dr. Fred Lee, patients treated with hormonal therapy before surgery had a lower incidence of positive margins (cancer growth outside the prostate) than the surgery only group (8 percent versus 34 percent, respectively). The seminal vesicles are routinely removed during this operation since it is one of the first areas to which cancer spreads.

Dr. Hricak, Professor of Radiology at Cornell Medical Center, noted a review of post surgical MRI exams showed part or all of the seminal vesicles remained postoperatively in 57 percent of cases in the study. This begs the question: Why not perform an MRI or sonogram before finishing the operation to ensure these organs have been completely removed and ensure that this potential area of cancer spread is no longer a threat.

Radiation therapy, using external beam procedures, usually takes seven weeks, with treatments five days a week. Each treatment takes about 10 minutes. Radiation is beamed through healthy tissues to the diseased prostate. Complications of external beam radiation are: incontinence 10 percent, impotence 29-49 percent, urinary obstruction 10 percent and irritable bowel problems 8 percent. Recovery is up to 2 months after the full course of treatment. Cancer may recur in 30–50 percent. The 2006 American Urologic Association meeting featured a study by Dr. Albertsen following men treated by surgery, radiation and watchful waiting. Of interest in this non randomized study, it was noted that there was no difference in survival between radiation and watchful waiting. IMRT or Intensity Modulated Radiation Therapy using computerized targeting seems to have fewer side effects but may involve up to 45 treatments over a course of nine weeks. Proton therapy, performed at only a handful of major cancer treatment centers, may prove more useful, although I had a patient with a massive recurrence only 6 months following treatment. It should be noted that radiated tissue is very fragile and treating a recurrent tumor by any modality involves increased risk. Most significantly, according to the 2006 *World Conference of Interventional Oncology* talk by senior radiation therapist, Dr. Thomas DiPetrillo, high grade prostate cancers respond poorly to any type of radiation therapy.

Complications of Brachytherapy or Internal Radiation Seeds, a permanent implantation of the 80–100 radioactive pellets in the prostate, are: impotence 20 percent, rectal problems 5 percent, migration of seeds to lungs in 36 percent of patients and prolonged urinary symptoms in many cases. Cancer may recur in 20 percent. The 2006 World Congress of Interventional Oncology presented papers demonstrating that radiation therapy was least effect for patients with high grade tumors.

At this point I will insert the significant findings of the 2007 Meeting of Radiation Therapists at the NY Roentgen Society National Prostate Cancer Symposium:

PSA: Usually decreases during successful treatment over a six month time period. Increases may be due to local or distant tumor spread.

BIOPSY: 20–30% of successfully treated tumors that are biochemically stable (low PSA) have cancer discovered on repeat biopsies after one or two years.

TREATMENT WITH IMRT: Higher dose results in fewer post treatment positive biopsies but result in higher rates of incontinence and impotence. Higher dose may double the incidence of secondary cancers in long term survivors. There is a trend to reduce side effects by offering focal treatment-that is, treating only the cancerous tissue and sparing the remaining normal prostate gland. Emphasis on proper positioning of the beam due to motion of the prostate gland was discussed. Since the gland can move up to 1 cm (1/3 inch), the targeting is adjusted by CT or ultrasound scans of the prostate before treatment. Most tumors are in the periphery of the prostate so it is essential that this area lie in the central treatment beam.

FUTURE DEVELOPMENTS: Several speakers thought the introduction of power Doppler imaging would be useful to focus the beam on the most aggressive area while sparing the benign tissue or lower grade tumor. This modality could also be used to detect local recurrence. The 3D capability could adjust the beam to compensate for prostate motion.

Complications of cryosurgery, a minimally invasive freezing of the prostate tissues, are: Incontinence 5 percent, impotence 85 percent, urinary obstruction 10 percent. Recovery is 2 days. Cancer may recur in 15 percent. A variation of cryosurgery called "partial cryotherapy" has fewer side effects.

Complications of HIFU (high intensity focused ultrasound), minimally invasive use of intersecting, computer focused ultrasound waves to ablate diseased tissue, are: incontinence 1 percent, impotence 5 percent. Recovery includes a catheter worn for 2–4 weeks. Resumption of normal lifestyle starts immediately. Cancer may recur in 16 percent. Recurrent tumor may be re-treated by the HIFU procedure or other therapies.

Complications of RFA, internal heating of small (less than 1 inch/ 3 cm tumors) tumors by radio waves, are: incontinence 0 percent, impotence 0 percent. There is a possibility of a tract created between urethra and rectum. Recovery is immediate, if local anesthesia is used. There is no data on cancer recurrence available on this new procedure.

A fuller discussion of the minimally invasive procedures of cryosurgery (freezing), RFA (cooking) and HIFU (heating) is appropriate due to current FDA approval policies. Medicare approved Cryosurgery in 2001 to treat the recurrent cancer that occurs in 25 percent of radiation treated patients. Seventy-three percent of patients treated with Targeted Cryosurgery after failing radiation showed no signs of cancer at 4 years, according to Dr. Douglas Chinn, a pioneer in this field. Cryosurgery may be repeated if cancer recurs. Specimens examined from radical surgical prostatectomy often indicate that cancer has already spread outside the gland (positive surgical margin), meaning that the operation did not remove the cancer completely. It has been reported that 50 percent of radical procedures demonstrate a positive surgical margin and that radiation therapy has a 50 percent failure rate after 5 years. Cryotherapy has emerged as an effective alternative to these treatments.

Cryosurgery, also called cryotherapy or cryoablation, of the prostate involves controlled freezing of the gland to destroy both cancerous and native prostatic tissues. The early high rate of complications was reduced by improvements in ultrasound guided imaging systems. This treatment is generally performed under spinal or general anesthesia. Dr. D. Bahn published a seven year series where the biopsy proven disease-free-rate was 85.8 percent. While the technique has the advantages of being minimally invasive, repeatable if necessary and cost effective, the disadvantages are that there have been no long term randomized multi-center studies. Also, like most ultrasound guided therapies, the procedure is highly operator dependent, implying the practicing physician must have significant experience with many cases.

The other repeatable procedure is the HIFU ablation. Repeat RFA has not yet been performed due to the short time this has been clinically available. While HIFU has fewer side effects, so far, it is not approved by the FDA and is currently being performed outside the United States. The procedure may not be covered or reimbursed by US insurance companies. A report from the French Institute of Health and Medical Research in Paris showed stated "Focused pulses of ultrasound can eradiate prostate cancer as effective as cutting the tumor out with surgery, but often with far fewer side effects" as quoted in the March 2004 issue of *Urology*. In order to reduce the side effects of urinary retention, Drs. Christian Chaussy and Stefan Thuroff, from Munich, perform a TURP to reduce prostate volume. Results of a European multicenter trial, published in the 2003 Journal of Endourology by Drs. Thuroff, Chaussy and Vallancien, stated that this procedure was safe and may be useful as a primary therapy for prostate cancer. Drs. Ethan Halpern and Barry Goldberg, authors of the current radiology textbook *IMAGING OF THE PROSTATE,* from Thomas Jefferson University Hospital, note the HIFU ablation of cancer presents a competitive alternative to conventional surgical treatment. In their article in the 2005 Journal *RADIOLOGY* they say, "The ability to focus and accurately target a lesion with high intensity focused ultrasound by using ultra-sound or MRI guidance allows precise ablation of lesions of any shape without damage to surrounding structures."

A new procedure for the treatment of the prostate is radiofrequency ablation (RFA) whereby heat generated by radio waves destroys cancers. Radio waves produce internal heating that coagulates the tissues. As a US Air Force radiologist from 1970–72, I saw injuries in the airmen stationed in Greenland warming themselves by standing in front of the radar antennae. The inner warmth they felt was their internal organs being cooked just like micro-waved food by the high energy radio waves. This FDA approved procedure has been successfully performed for many years on breast, liver and kidney cancers in the US and has recently been successfully performed on the prostate in European trials. The side effect, that is partially avoidable, is damage to the rectum. This sensitive area is monitored carefully by temperature probes in all the minimally invasive procedures. A 2006 study published in *PROSTATE CANCER AND PROSTATIC DISEASES* by Dr. F. Bergamaschi, a urologist from the University Hospital in Milan, Italy has shown this modality to kill tumors with pin point accuracy.

In 2003 I learned about HIFU on the prostate at a medical seminar in Miami. I decided to check it out and flew down to the Dominican Republic. HIFU was considered a novel therapeutic tool since the 1940's and was used successfully in brain surgery in the 1960's. In the early 1990's, initial work on the prostate was targeted at benign prostatic hypertrophy (BPH). From 1992-93, the first group of cancer patients was treated at the Indiana University School of Medicine. Since then, the Japanese, Germans, Canadians and French have used HIFU treatments as an approved technology.

I accompanied one of my patients who had independently chosen to undergo this procedure as his primary definitive treatment. I, herewith, recount my initial personal experience with this modality: After spinal anesthesia, which eliminates pain and prevents movement of the lower body and keeps the gland motionless, an ultrasound probe is placed in the rectum similar to the standard diagnostic transrectal ultrasound (TRUS) exam. The prostate is scanned. A computer map is made of the gland and the tumor, including the adjacent seminal vesicles to which cancer frequently spreads. The targeting of the tumor takes 5–10 minutes. The treating portion of the machine then takes about 20–30 minutes to sequentially destroy a volume of the prostate tissue. This is repeated until all the organ has been targeted and treated. As the treating probe coagulates the prostatic tissues, the dark colored cancer on the screen turns white with every 2 mm sweep of the beam.

The physician monitors the procedure, which is electromechanically automated and computer driven, and adjusts it as needed to steer the beam clear of the rectal wall or to deliver ablative energy to a portion of the tumor that has penetrated through the capsule. This HIFU technology is currently being performed in Japan, Mexico, Canada and Europe and is currently undergoing phase III trials in the United States.

My patient's treatment, start to finish, took three hours. He went home the next morning. Two weeks later he removed his catheter and was fully recovered and symptom free. He was extraordinarily happy, since his neighbor was just getting out of the hospital from having prostate radical surgery at the same time his HIFU ablation occurred. The HIFU technology is made by EDAP Technomed in Europe and is slightly different from the American made equipment by USHIFU. I have since reported my 3 years experience with HIFU at the 2006 JFR

Meeting, my 4 years experience at the 2007 ARRS and 2007 ICS Meetings which confirm the earlier stated findings.

Another patient, Robert B, a North Carolina native, reports his HIFU experience as follows in a fax dated June 20, 2005:

In 2000 at the age of 67 I had my first PSA test taken during a physical. It was 7.4 and the Dr. advised me to see a urologist as soon as possible. I had a biopsy and an ultrasound which was negative. My PSA was rising at each 6 month Drs. Visit. In December, 2003, I had a positive biopsy and a PSA reading of 16.2. I decided to go on a diet of supplements and fasting for a complete body cleanse. This seemed to stop the PSA from rising temporarily, then it rose to 17.4 and I realized something had to be done. My urologist recommended hormone treatments, seeding with radioactive pellets and radiation beam treatment. I did not want to go this route. In April 2004 a herbalist recommended Dr. Bard in NYC who had a power Doppler 3D imaging ultrasound system. I saw Dr. Bard in May of 2004 and he found I did not have aggressive cancer at that time. However, in 5 months it became aggressive. He gave me several options to choose from and I decided on the High Intensity Focused Ultrasound (HIFU). In December 2004 I went to the Dominican Republic for the non invasive procedure. It went very well. In April 2005 the PSA was down to 7.4. The vascular tumor is no longer present and there is a marked decrease in prostate volume. The prognosis is excellent and life once again has meaning.

Technicalities aside, the main clinical advantage of the USHIFU brand called Sonablate 500 is that the imaging and treatment probes are in one unit. This allows the physician to simultaneously image and treat. This ensures that the treatment areas have not changed by patient movement (voluntarily or involuntarily as in coughing, bowel motions, etc). In fact, the tissue changes accompanying treatment are noted in the moment. The high energy sound waves are focused into a small area creating intense heat of 80–100 degrees Centigrade. This temperature is lethal to prostate cancer. The tissues outside the focal zone are not injured by the sound waves. Specifically, tissues 2 mm away from the thermal delivery dose are not injured in the 1 second pulse of energy that kills the targeted area. In time the treated organ regresses in size as it is eliminated by the body's natural disposal systems.

Dr. Douglas Chinn, in the February 2005 issue of PCRI Insights, feels any patient with organ confined prostate cancer is a primary candidate for this procedure. He notes the advantages of HIFU because it can treat the tumor that has begun to spread beyond the prostate capsule, and if it has not spread beyond the capsule and the neurovascular bundles (nerves) are not involved, then the nerves can be spared and potency maintained.

This is an e mail of a patient dated 6-27-05:

In October of 2004 I went to see my internist for a routine annual physical. He was the chief of staff at our local hospital and had won my trust over the preceding 30 years as an excellent diagnostician and very competent clinician. As usual, my physical exam was without incident. He took a blood sample and ordered the usual tests with one exception. This time he ordered the usual PSA test plus a second test which measured something he called "free PSA." As he said, "Now that you've turned 60, let's throw in this fairly new test for free PSA levels and see how you look. I wasn't terribly worried because my PSA scores had been within clinical limits in the past, and because his physical exam revealed nothing. This procedure was being ordered because my doctor was a cautious and learned sort of man, watching over his patients rather diligently.

He called the next week to tell me that all test results were normal.... except the free PSA results. Then he said something he had never said to me in 30 years—"I'm concerned. Please see your urologist for further testing." Anxiety immediately set in, but it was limited by my awareness that PSA tests were notoriously unreliable.

One week later I saw a urologist and one week after that he told me in his office that my internist was right, my free PSA scores were elevated to the point that I had a 20-25% chance of having prostate cancer. He then explained that free PSA testing originated with a medical researcher who had shown in two different studies that free PSA was a very useful indicator for possible prostate cancer. He added that he was most impressed by my internist since he was sure that no more than a handful of internists in our area were even aware of the test. I barely heard what he said. I had gone into a world of worst case scenarios. When I finally came back to the conversation he was recommending that I get an ultra sound exam t his second office and, if necessary, a biopsy. Possible treatments would not be discussed until and unless cancer was found. I stumbled my way out of his office, made an appointment to see him for an ultra sound test in one week, and drove home.

Though shaken I kept reminding myself that a 25% chance of cancer meant that I had a 75% chance of not having cancer. As the time for his ultrasound test drew near I called the president of our county's prostate self-help group. His advice was simple: "If I was going to have an ultra sound, I would go to the best. So I cancelled my appointment with my urologist and made an appointment with Dr. Bard.

I tried to stay calm in Dr. Bard's examining room, with limited success. However, pure terror took over when Dr. Bard located the actual cancerous tumor with his ultra sound machine. I strained to remember what I had decided in Dr. Bard's waiting room. After reviewing the numbers on different types of cancer treatments, I had decided that if Dr. Bard's examination was positive for cancer I would opt for high intensity ultra sound treatment, HIFU. HIFU had the best cure rate and the least probability for incontinence and impotence. It scared me to opt for something that was not offered in the USA, and it scared me to select a cancer treatment which I had not read about in the New England Journal of Medicine. HIFU had not been approved for prostate cancer in the USA. However, HIFU had been used for other problems in the USA. I believe gallstones or something like that. It has also been used with prostate cancer for years in Europe. In fact, the final, though not primary, factor in my decision was that I had somehow heard of HIFU many years earlier in some dimly remembered medical paper or discussion, and I remember thinking at the time, "Boy, if I ever got cancer, that would be the way to go."

However, the next step was to get another opinion from a radiologist using an MRI. I was so upset and scared that Dr. Bard's office staff took pity on me, mobilized and arranged an MRI appointment for me one hour later. That, too, was positive for cancer. Dr. Bard studied his three dimensional images for a long time after the MRI, making sure he was convinced that the tumor had not breached the prostate wall and that I was a candidate for HIFU. Once he declared HIFU could be used in my case, his office staff, with plaintive entreaties from me, mobilized around my terror once again. They contacted the office of Dr. Suarez, a surgeon-urologist who practiced HIFU for cancer treatment outside of the USA. Within ten minutes I was scheduled for a HIFU intervention approximately nine days later. I was determined to act and to act quickly and decisively, especially after Dr, Bard noted that the tumor had lots of blood supply and was likely to be very active. At least, that it was I concluded after looking at the ultrasound pictures and hearing Dr. Bard say. "If it were me, I would address this in less than three to six months." Nine days was within those parameters, much to my relief.

On the weekend before Thanksgiving of 2004, my wife and I flew to Mexico where I was to undergo the HIFU procedure. I was treated caringly, though any slight divergence from expectation put me into an intense worrisome state. To get to the heart of the matter, Dr. Suarez demolished my cancerous tumor with his extraordinarily precise HIFU machine. I was comforted by the fact that five or six urologists were in attendance, watching Dr. Suarez perform this procedure. I am told that it took two or three hours, but I don't know whether that was because the HIFU procedure takes that long, or because Dr, Suarez was explaining, teaching and answering questions from the other five or six urologists who were present. I was told I talked non-stop through the entire procedure and that all present knew my life history from my non-stop monologue, but I don't remember that. The anesthesiologist, who was quite kind to me, had done such a good job that I was spared all pain and all anxiety. In fact, from the moment the anesthesiologist and I had such a pleasant and warm-hearted chat, until the time he was telling me that I could soon return to the hotel when I was staying, I only have two memories. The first was turning to Dr. Suarez just before the anesthesia kicked in and saying, "Get it all no matter what it takes." The second was Dr. Suarez appearing and saying to me "It's done. I got it all."

One hour later I was back at the hotel where I and the HIFU staff, including Dr. Suarez were staying. The next day I flew home with a catheter in and, hopefully, the cancer out. I was now with my entire family, telling my three children that I was going to be fine. Two days later I was back at the work I love. I saw my internist for that first fateful visit in mid-October 2004. I flew home from Mexico after receiving the HIFU procedure or intervention in mid-November, just in time for Thanksgiving. The entire experience took slightly more than a month. Watchful waiting, prolonged thoughtful investigations, family discussions and specialist debates were definitely not for me. One month was about the length of time that I could hold up, so I'm thrilled and grateful that Dr. Bard made it happen.

At home I followed the post-procedure protocol, took the appropriate medications, had my catheter removed, used a diaper for a short time, particularly on trips or when I was going to exercise, discovered to my great relief that I was not incontinent, and then, slowly, discovered that I was not impotent. If I lived, it was going to be as a fairly normal man.

Three months later I saw Dr. Bard. I was completely overjoyed when he confirmed Dr. Suarez' remark, "I got it all." I thanked Dr, Bard for saving my life, for without him who knows what would have happened. I cannot imagine anything producing the kind of result I got without the severe side effects that are all too common with men who have cancer of the prostate.

The story has one small sequel. About six months after the HIFU procedure, I noticed that my urine stream was slowing. This went on for several weeks. I ignored it, figuring it was nothing special, perhaps a small infection. Then my urine flow slowed to the point that I could scarcely urinate. I was not comfortable gong back to the urologist I had used way back in November, assuming he would look most unfavorably on my choice to bypass his aid in favor of a new procedure not even authorized by the FDA. I called Dr. Bard, who once again gave me the right person, a urologist who had trained half of the urologists in NYC. I went to see him expecting to be told that my bladder was distended or my prostate was swollen or something like that. All my organs checked out fine. He took a culture to see *if I was struggling with an infection still. However, he hypothesized that something, perhaps the HIFU procedure, had caused my to tighten all the muscles involved with urination. He prescribed Flomax. It didn't seem to work. By now all urine flow had completely ceased, no matter how much water I drank. I called my new urologist. He told me to meet him at his office in one hour. Just as I was about to leave the house, I tried one last "technique." I bent over repeatedly to tie my shoes. On the sixth try I felt a "pop." Urine came gushing out as I made my way to the toilet in haste. Some strange looking particle appeared in my toilet. I fished it out, not knowing whether it had been there all day or had been deposited there by the urinary flood that just erupted. I saved it in a jar. Over the next week or two, several more particles appeared. I saved them and brought them to my urologist. He sent them to the lab. When I visited him to find out about the results of the culture and of the specimen examination he informed me that I was infection free but that something had happened that he had never seen before in 35 years of practice, teaching and supervision. Now I was scared. I saw a report from the lab complete with colored charts. Then he explained: "you have pissed out your prostate." Necrotic, infected prostatic tissue had been blocking my urinary passage.*

Sure enough, days later Dr. Bard showed pictures to me demonstrating the truth of the lab report and the urologist's statement. In the three months between my first post-HIFU ultrasound and this second one, a significant portion of my prostate had disappeared, or in the vernacular, been "pissed out." Dr. Suarez had told me that the prostate would disintegrate in the 12 months following the HIFU procedure, but I don't think he expected anything this dramatic.

However, this mattered not one bit to me. I was rendered ecstatic once again by Dr. Bard's second ultrasound exam which showed no living cancer cells in my prostate. God willing, it will stay that way. But if any problem pops up, I will absolutely follow Dr. Bard's advice.

One of the disadvantages of thermal therapies is that the destroyed prostatic tissue may exit the body by the urinary tract and cause temporary obstruction to the urethra. While this is a relatively minor side effect and can be remedied with the insertion of a small catheter and irrigation with fluid, it must be mentioned as another delayed type complication of HIFU, cryosurgery and RFA. Scarring of the prostatic urethra resulting in decreased urine flow may require a surgical procedure to dilate this area at some point in time. While some physicians attempt to eliminate this problem by performing a TURP to open up the urethra before the HIFU treatment, I have noted several cases of incontinence in patients with only minimal prostatic enlargement.

Another use of HIFU is in salvage therapy, meaning that recurrent cancer after radiation therapy or surgery may be re-treated. Dr. Chinn, who has patented temperature monitoring technology and trains physicians in cryosurgery, feels HIFU will be better for salvage therapy than cryosurgery because of the excellent targeting of tissue. Contra-indications to HIFU are extensively calcified glands because sound waves are blocked by calcium and rectal stenosis where the probe cannot be inserted into the anus. Similar to cryosurgery, bleeding disorders are not absolute contra-indications. Blood thinners should be stopped 10 days in advance because there may be rectal bleeding due to the probe insertion that causes stretching of the bowel wall.

The long term results USHIFU presented at the 2005 National Conference on Prostate Cancer in Washington DC are the five year disease free (by PSA testing) survival rates of the five most widely used invasive prostate cancer local treatments, and this reveals that HIFU results compare well with the results of these other therapies, while demonstrating low side effects. With the new Sonablate system, the rectal injury rate has been reduced from 5 percent to less than 0.5 percent. Dr. Thuroff from Munich presented his study of 1000 cases treated with the EDAP HIFU system at the 100th Annual American Urological Association Meeting showing high patient acceptance and excellent clinical results in patients with localized prostate cancer. A French study by Dr. A. Gelet presented at the same conference evaluated the 5 year results of HIFU treatment in a population of 230 patients. He concluded with this "minimally invasive treatment is related to an acceptable morbidity rate and a high local control of the localized prostate cancer. The treatment's repeatability remains a unique advantage of this option." A recent change from the penile catheter to a suprapublic (bladder) catheter has allowed for a smoother postoperative course and quicker recovery.

The prestigious university hospital in Paris, Hopital Necker Infante Malades with the largest urology department in France, is using RFA to treat kidney tumors this year and will begin utilizing this technique on prostate cancers in 2008. RFA appears to be useful for smaller tumors in the prostate. Dr. Antonio Giorgio of the Interventional Ultrasound Service of Cotugno Hospital in Italy has developed a needle electrode that adds salt solution to the treatment site, which increases the effectiveness and decreases side effects. In his article published in the 2005 *American Journal of Radiology,* he reports that his three year study in his work with liver tumors has had few side effects and is considered safe. Currently, RFA is being performed clinically in Milan and Frankfurt.

Other disorders apparent on the 3-D PDS are: Benign prostatic hyperplasia (benign overgrowth), prostatitis (acute infection), abscess (pocket of pus), chronic infection (prostatitis and tuberculosis), stones (like gallstones and kidney stones) and bladder tumors. Diseases related to prostate cancer outside the prostate partially amenable to evaluation by 3-D PDS are lymphadenopathy (malignant glands), vascular metastases (tumor spread to bone and liver), ascites (malignant fluid build up) and rectal wall invasion (tumor extending into the bowel).

WATCHFUL WAITING / ACTIVE SURVEILLANCE

Dr. Laurence Klotz, Professor of Surgery at the University of Toronto, in the 2006 PCRI INSIGHTS article makes the following observations and recommendations about low grade prostate cancer:

- 50–60% of patients fall into the risk category acceptable for active surveillance
- 10% mortality of untreated Gleason 6 at 20 years
- 80–100 radical prostatectomies are required for each PC death averted
- Eligibility for active surveillance:
    PSA < 11   Gleason <7   Biopsy cores positive <4 and <50% of core

- Follow up schedule:
    PSA/DRE every 3 months for 2 years
    10–12 core biopsy at one year/then every 3–5 years till age 80

- Intervention when:
    PSA doubles in 3 years / Gleason 7 on rebiopsy

I do not make treatment recommendations. Instead, I give my patients the full range of facts and let them choose their therapy. Together we then monitor their progress. The treatment programs below are the most popular therapeutic pathways that patients have chosen. Patients seem to prefer quality of life to quantity of life. Many understand that a reasonable lifestyle made possible by controlling a disease with few treatment side effects is preferable to curing a medical problem with life altering consequences of the therapy. In other words, the treatment should not be worse than the cure.

A friend's dog had to have a front leg amputated due to a car accident. We were worried how the dog would react to the trauma of the disfigurement and the inability to walk as before. We even joked about canine psychotherapy. Upon removal of the cast, Rover, as he was called, took a step and fell. Rover repositioned his remaining foreleg to the center and proceeded to walk without discomfort. Another animal example was of a homeless cat who was wandering the street. An animal lover took the cat home to give better care and turn him into a pet. The male cat took an instant dislike to his new surroundings and made the house unlivable. Within a week he was returned to the street where he resumed his preferred, if nomadic, living arrangements. This analogy supports the idea that the end result must be acceptable to the lifestyle.

Another patient was a former high fashion model who had fractured her arm skiing. When the cast was taken off, x-rays showed bone fragments within the elbow joint prohibiting full range of motion. The surgeon suggested replacing the joint with a new plastic and metallic device that would restore full motion. After the operation, 8 weeks of physical therapy would be required. My patient chose to use the other arm for tasks requiring full mobility and the injured arm for less active chores. Similarly, men with urinary frequency can choose to drink less water when they go for long car rides or plane trips.

Patients with no biopsy or a negative biopsy and a normal 3-D PDS, choose a repeat exam in one year. Supplements for the prostate are recommended. If there is a family history of cancer, a six month follow-up scan is usually performed. These days, as the emergence of "interval cancers" is better appreciated, for peace of mind, men are choosing to be screened on a six month rotation.

This is the half year time period health conscious women choose to alert themselves to the possibility of early breast cancer as they routinely undergo ultrasound breast screening twice a year. In my practice 5 percent of men develop aggressive interval cancers within half a year from their last normal or stable evaluation. Indeed, one of my female patients left on vacation with the peace of mind from just having a normal mammogram and sonogram to spend a month vacationing in San Diego. There she discovered a new lump which repeated mammograms and sonograms proved to be a 2 cm (2/3 inch) new cancer which had developed in only four weeks. This extreme example authenticates the recommendation of half yearly screening for interval cancers. A presentation *INTERVAL CANCERS OF THE PROSTATE: EVALUATION BY 3-T MRI AND 3-D POWER DOPPLER ULTRASOUND* was presented at the 2006 meeting of the Societe Francaise de Radiologie in Paris demonstrating that new aggressive tumors may occur more rapidly than clinically expected and may, in part, explain the failure of certain treatments.

Patients having a positive biopsy in only a few segments of low grade cancer with the majority of the biopsies showing no tumor and no evidence of high-grade cancer on 3-D PDS, choose a six-month follow-up scan. Treatment alternatives are: watchful waiting with supplements, HIFU, localized cryosurgery or focal radio frequency ablation (RFA) of a localized cancer.

When a man has not had a biopsy or has had a negative biopsy and a vascular tumor is demonstrated on the 3-D PDS, I perform an MRI exam, which shows the prostate gland, the capsule of the prostate, the regional lymph glands, seminal vesicles and boney pelvis. Other bones, to which cancer frequently spreads such as the lower spine and hip, may also be imaged for abnormalities. While the MRI exam is not as good an indicator of cancer aggression, it shows spread of the tumor outside the prostate capsule to the lymph nodes better then the 3-D PDS and better than the CT scan, which is currently used as the standard test for staging.

The radioisotope or nuclear scan has had too many false positives and negatives and may go the way of the PSA exam. I have several patients who come in yearly who had diagnosed prostate cancer with positive findings on the nuclear isotope scan over twelve years ago who are doing well without clinical evidence of this disease. One patient was even told he would be dead within six months—that was 18 years ago when the isotope scan showed "metastases" to the spine. Given the natural history of cancer in the prostate and the complications of biopsy, men prefer the 3-D PDS/MRI exam combination instead of the biopsy. Indeed, many patients and most non-surgical physicians fear that the cutting of the tumor will spread the cancer locally throughout the biopsy site and distantly, as malignant cells spread into the blood stream to different areas. Patients with vascular tumors choose alternative treatments for 3 months and rescan for follow up evaluation with the 3-D PDS. If the vascularity is unchanged or decreased, treatment is continued for a 4-month period and the patient again rescanned. If there are no interval changes, scans continue every 6 months. Unfortunately, biopsies have missed significant cancers in patients that are imaged by 3D-PDS and MRI. Since 2000, the American College of Radiology has recommended yearly that the area of high vascularity be the primary target for biopsy. Few urologists have the sophisticated equipment or extensive training and experience to perform this study today. According to a *Miami Herald* article, January 2004, most of the patients who forgo a needle biopsy and head directly to non invasive treatment are physicians themselves.

Patients with a positive biopsy and a high grade tumor on the 3-D PDS often choose HIFU, cryosurgery or RFA, if the tumor is organ confined, that is, retained within the prostate gland, and there is no evidence of distant spread. Reduction of the tumor mass is often first attempted by use of hormones or high intensity alternative therapies, after which another definitive treatment is considered. Radiation is considered if these protocols are not possible for a particular reason. Data presented at the JFR 2006 and WCIO 2006 support the use of high intensity anti oxidant treatments and many anecdotal reports of tumor stabilization and regression are noted. A treatise by me at the JFR 2006 details 99 men with high grade cancers treated solely by diet, plant sterols and antioxidants with 90% effectiveness in local tumor control within 3 to 6 months.

PARTIAL CRYOSURGERY

Gary Onik MD from the Center for Surgical Advancement, Departments of Radiology and Urology, Celebration Health/Florida Hospital in Celebration, Florida presented an article called "Rationale for a Male Lumpectomy," A Prostate Cancer Targeted Approach Using Cryoablation at the 2005 American Roentgen Ray Society Meeting. He feels the use of breast sparing surgery i.e., "lumpectomy," to treat breast cancer has revolutionized management of that disease. Lumpectomy showed that the quality of life of the patients can successfully be integrated into the equation of cancer treatment without compromising treatment efficacy. Prostate cancer in men raises many of the same issues that breast cancer does in women. Complications of prostate cancer treatments, including impotence and incontinence, affect the male self-image and psyche no less than a woman's loss of a breast does. Pathologic literature indicates that up to 35 percent of prostate cancers are solitary and unilateral. This raises the question of whether these patients can be identified and treated with a limited "lumpectomy". His paper presents a pilot study in which 21 patients were treated with a focal cryoablation procedure. Focal cryoablation was performed if the tumor was confined to only one prostate lobe.

Cryoablation was planned to encompass the area of the known tumor. Patients obtained PSA's every 3 months for two years and then every 6 months thereafter. Follow-up ranged from 24–105 months with a mean of 50 months. Twenty of 21 (95 percent) patients had stable PSA's with no evidence for cancer, despite 10 patients being medium to high risk for recurrence. All 19 patients had a biopsy to detect recurrent cancer were negative. Seventeen of the 21 patients (80 percent) maintained their potency. No other complications, including incontinence or fistula formation, were noted. He concluded that these results indicate a "male lumpectomy" in which the prostate tumor region itself is destroyed, sparing the rest of the gland, preserving potency in a majority of patients and limiting other complications without compromising cancer control- is a viable option. If confirmed by further studies and long term follow-up, this treatment approach could have a profound effect on prostate cancer management.

Dr. Onik, a pioneer in cryosurgery, has based his theory on a number of recent studies that have questioned the efficacy of an aggressive treatment approach to prostate cancer. Current management of prostate cancer covers both ends of the treatment spectrum. Patients can elect no treatment at all i.e. "watchful waiting" or aggressive whole gland treatments, such as radical prostatectomy with no middle ground available. It stands to reason that if no treatment at all can be advocated for a subset of prostate cancer patients, then the compromise of attempting to just destroy the focus of cancer in the gland could be a viable option. Cryoablation, using imaging guidance, unlike traditional treatments such as radical prostatectomy and radiation, is technically, very well suited to a "lumpectomy" type approach.

The main theoretical objection to a lumpectomy type approach to prostate cancer is the realization that prostate cancer is often a multi-focal disease within the prostate. As in breast cancer, however, prostate cancer is a spectrum of diseases, some of which may be amenable to lumpectomy and others that may not. The prostate cancer pathology literature clearly shows that many patients do not have multi-focal prostate cancer. Until now, however, little attention has been paid in trying to differentiate those patients with unifocal from multi-focal disease; the reason for this is that it had little clinical significance, when treatments were all aimed at total gland removal or destruction.

A study examining radical prostatectomy specimens showed that patients with unifocal disease constituted one third of the cases studied and could be reliably differentiated from patients with multi-focal disease with a sensitivity of 90 percent using the PSA test. In addition, 80 percent of multi-focal tumors are less than 0.5 cc's, indicating they may not be of clinical significance. Drs. Rukstalis and Noguchi confirmed this study in which pathologic examination showed that uni-focal tumors were present in 25 percent of patients. Using the size criteria of 5 mm or less as an insignificant tumor, an additional 60 percent and 39 percent of patients might be a candidate for a focal treatment approach. Clearly then, based on the known pathology of prostate cancer an opportunity exists to investigate a lumpectomy type approach. The question has to be raised—if these patients with unifocal disease can be clinically identified? It has been demonstrated that optimization of biopsy results by a second set of biopsies and improved gland sampling can greatly diminish the chances of missing a significant multi-focal tumor.

The anatomy of the prostate does not make it accessible to surgical lumpectomy; tumor destruction by another modality is needed to realize a lumpectomy in a male. Physicians chose cryoablation because it has a long history of effective tumor treatment in various parts of the body. The early rocky start that prostate cryoablation experienced has been largely mitigated by major technical advances in the procedure, such as improved urethral warmer design, and has been shown to be an effective and safe alternative in treating the prostate cancer involving the gwhole gland. Drs. Donnelly and Bahn recently published long term data confirming cryoablation is a competitive treatment to both surgery and radiation in treating prostate cancer. Dr. Katz and colleagues recently published article reviews the 5 year biochemical disease free survival of patients treated with brachytherapy, CT conformal radiation therapy, radical prostatectomy and cryoablation for every article published in the last 10 years. The results were stratified based on whether the patients were low, medium or high risk for biochemical failure. Based on this analysis the range of results for cryoablation was equivalent to all other treatments in low and medium risk patients and appeared to be superior in high risk patients. Overall complications rates were similar with all the modalities. Dr. Gould published the only article directly comparing cryoablation with radical prostatectomy. It showed cryoablation to be equivalent to radical prostatectomy (RP) in low risk patients but as patient's preoperative PSA increased, cryoablation results were superior to RP. The basis for this apparent superiority in high risk patients may be the ability of cryoablation to treat extra-capsular extension of cancer and to be repeated without any additional morbidity, if needed. Based on these results, one can conclude that cryoablation is a safe and effective treatment for treating prostate cancer, and its inherent ability to be tailored to the extent of a patient's disease, makes it a platform upon which a treatment such as lumpectomy can be based.

Dr. Onik's earlier results previously reported in the journal *Urology* and in the 2005 American Roentgen Ray Meeting noted that patients with unifocal prostate cancer could be successfully identified and treated with limited cryoablation. The additional patients and longer follow-up presented in this paper confirm the earlier results. Within the context of a follow-up of approximately 4 years, this approach has been successful in local cancer control and equivalent to the results cited for whole gland cryotherapy, as has been evidenced in stable PSA results in 95 percent of patients and negative postoperative biopsies in all 19 patients.

Lastly, known areas of potential extra capsular extension can be prophylactically treated by extending the freezing to encompass the peri-prostatic tissue in the area of the neurovascular bundle and seminal vesicles. This locally extensive freezing, which makes this procedure a unique combination of an aggressive yet conservative treatment, is facilitated by the technical advance of injecting saline solution into the soft tissues that separate the rectum from the prostate. Increasing this space eliminates the chance for rectal damage allowing greater freezing into extra-capsular regions.

The two major treatment side effects that prostate cancer patients fear the most are impotence and incontinence. Certainly, any minimally invasive prostate cancer treatment must minimize the incidence of these complications if it is to claim an advantage over the present whole gland treatments. By having extremely low morbidity, the procedure appears to fulfill the goal of a lumpectomy type procedure. None of the patients had significantly long-term incontinence after the procedure with all but one patient who became fully continent immediately.

Unfortunately, radiation therapy does not appear to maintain its initial potency advantage over the long term. Potency rates after 2 years are essentially equivalent with nerve sparing radical prostatectomy. The use of radioactive seeds (brachytherapy) causes urinary tract complications and can have a significant effect on patient lifestyle. And, rectal complications, a major concern with radiation therapy, have been virtually eliminated in this procedure by separation of the rectum and prostate with saline injection prior to freezing. In addition, brachytherapy patients who fail locally have limited curative options available. Lastly, a major drawback to radiation therapy is that patients who fail radiation show a significant increase in Gleason grade, and tumor aggressiveness in the recurrent cancer adversely effect patient survival. Certainly, this is not a favorable characteristic in a procedure being applied to possibly a younger patient population.

At present Dr. Onik is using cryoablation to carry out this cancer targeted treatment, since it has the demonstrated long term efficacy in treating prostate cancer. The important concept, however, is not which ablation technology is used but that a population of prostate cancer patients can be identified and successfully treated with a lumpectomy approach. Undoubtedly, if long term viability of such a treatment is demonstrated, then other forms of thermal ablation will be attempted such as RF, microwave and high intensity focused ultrasound, to accomplish the same end. A less satisfactory approach would be to attempt a focal treatment with radiation therapy, since the lack of real time feedback to guide therapy, the limitations of dose threshold and the inherent nature of radiation scatter, make it a less than optimal modality for this purpose. A new approach by Dr. Onik, called "electroporation" discussed cellular disruption technologies at the 2006 *First World Congress of Interventional Oncology.*

In 2004 I first met with Drs. Onik and Chinn, pioneers of cryotherapy and Dr. Suarez, an innovator of HIFU therapy to discuss the use of 3-D PDS to find focal cancer sites for "lumpectomy" treatments by these modalities. Our initial treatment and follow up results have been promising. I look forward to working in the future with Dr. Olivier Helenon, Director of the Radiology Department at Necker Hospital and Dr. Bertrand Dufour, Director of the Urology Department at Necker Hospital in Paris to pinpoint small tumors that will be part of a RFA multicenter international study. One of the unique benefits of RFA treatment is the ability to watch the abnormal blood vessels disappear completely after the procedure has finished giving the treating physician a definite endpoint. The ability of 3-D ultrasound to place the needle tip accurately into the center of the tumor on the first attempt has made the procedure quicker and more tolerable.

CHAPTER SEVEN

Assessing Response of Prostate Cancer Therapy

Standard medical practice suggests that the following are useful guides for evaluating the cancer's response to therapy:

- Clinical exam
- Imaging-CT, MRI, PET, 3D-PDS, isotope scans, PET/CT
- Tumor markers-PSA
- Performance status
- Sexual function
- Urinary function
- Quality of life
- Survival

The value of medical imaging is to:

- Determine efficacy of therapy
- Monitor changes
- Tailor future therapy
- Determine tumor recurrence
- Identify new tumor

One of the problems of evaluating cancer treatment is that the tumor may be rendered harmless or even dead but the volume of the tumor remains the same. That is, the cancer cells may be killed off and scar tissue replaces the dead cells, leaving the size of the original malignancy unchanged. This lesson was learned 10 years ago in treating liver tumors. The therapy would render the cancer harmless, but the size of the mass on the isotope scans, sonogram, CT and MRI would remain unchanged. The same is true of some prostate cancers that are inactivated but still feel like cancer on the digital rectal exam and show a mass effect on the sonogram and MRI. There needs to be a way to monitor changes and determine the efficacy of treatment. A common medical solution to this dilemma has been to obtain multiple needle biopsies 3 to 4 weeks after the procedure and look for cancer cells under the microscope. Fortunately, the blood flows in malignancies that have been inactivated decrease or disappear and can be quickly and accurately measured in the moment. Thus, with 3-D PDS there is a simple tool to quantify blood flow patterns to demonstrate therapeutic response. Dr. Bruno Fornage's 2005 study, published in *American Journal of Radiology,* showed that the blood flow in vascular tumors disappeared completely after fifteen minutes of RFA treatment providing an exact endpoint of the therapy. This feature is particularly useful in embolizing (blocking tumor blood vessels) vascular prostate disorders because the effect of the blockade shows immediately. If vessels were not properly occluded, the procedure can be repeated within minutes. The pathologist can see if the tumor has died and scarred down or turned into a benign jelly; however, the microscope cannot always tell that intact appearing cancers are inactivated and essentially harmless or possibly remain virulent and life threatening.

PET or Positron Emission Tomography, a nuclear isotope diagnostic tool has not been used much for evaluation of the prostate in the United States. A grant from the U.S. Department of Energy and the National Institute of Health to Japanese investigators Drs. Oyama and Akino showed new modifications may prove clinically useful. This work was presented at the 2005 American Urological Association Meeting. Likewise, a German study presented at the same meeting by Dr. Uwe Teiber showed PET was useful in detecting lymph node metastases better than CT scans and recommended further studies using the combination of PET/CT scanners. Yet another German group of urologists, Dr. Machtens and others, developed evidence that nuclear isotope scans with new generation radioactive tracers looked promising for the future as a prostate cancer detection tool. The physicians from the European cancer center in Ulm, Germany showed yet another nuclear isotope was useful in detecting local cancer recurrence. Dr. Bartsch concluded; "PET/CT is a promising diagnostic tool … able to demonstrate local lesions responsible for rising PSA … which could be verified by aimed transrectal ultrasound guided biopsy." In another paper at the AUA 2005 by Dr. Bartsch and colleagues, he reported 95% accuracy in detecting metastatic lymph nodes with PET/CT scans compared with operative findings. A paper by American radiologist in Texas, Dr. Joseph Basler and associates, following Dr. Bartsch's talk, showed that a Veteran's Administration study of the lymph node drainage of the prostate demonstrated a different path than expected. This presentation funded by the University of Texas Health Sciences Center cautioned "the current method of obturator node dissection with radical prostatectomy is inadequate and may explain a proportion of patients who fail local treatment despite adequate margin and traditional negative node status." A Swiss paper by Dr. D. Schmid presented in 2005 *RADIOLOGY,* recommended PET/CT for detecting local cancer recurrence and lymph node metastases. He recommended this test since MR detection of lymph node metastases had a low sensitivity and it has been shown that lymph node size does not correlate with the presence of prostate cancer metastases.

New MRI protocols to improve lymph node detection have been developed in the Netherlands by Dr. Jelle Barentsz, radiologist and President of the International Cancer Imaging Society. Pelvic lymph node metastases have a significant impact on the prognosis of patients with prostate cancer. Small lymph nodes involved with tumor spread means local treatments such as surgery and HIFU are not curative. Surgical lymph node detection has usually been performed by operative dissection of the pelvis. This was necessary since CT and MRI use size criteria to determine the presence or absence of disease. This means that nodes larger than 7 mm are suspicious but not definitive and may be due to inflammation or other non cancerous entities. Unfortunately, the prostate cancer tends to produce small areas called micrometastases that are often smaller than 7 mm. A new MRI technique using harmless iron oxide (rust) particles has shown to be 90% specific in predicting metastases and 98% specific in determining that there are no malignant areas. This requires a standard MRI and injection one day prior to the special MRI to observe abnormal lymph node areas. The test can detect tumor as small as 3 mm. A map of the malignant nodes is obtained which may be used for intensity modulated radiotherapy (IMRT). Diseased areas may be given more radiation and unaffected areas spared treatment. This work was presented at the 2006 *International Radiology Society* meeting.

What is the role of the Prostate Specific Antigen (PSA) in this scenario? The standards for the PSA are simple blood tests that look for high levels of an enzyme called prostate specific antigen, a potential warning sign of cancer. A number below 4 is considered normal. Men are usually advised to start getting this test yearly at age 50. Men with a family history of cancer are recommended to have this at an earlier age. Every man produces PSA, since it is the enzyme that helps break down fluids so that sperm can move more freely. For prostate screening, other PSA tests are also being studied. The usual test is called **Total PSA.** There also exist variations: Free PSA, Complex PSA, bPSA, iPSA and proPSA. Free PSA is often elevated due to benign problems. Complex PSA appears more specific for cancer. PSAV or PSA Velocity changes over time is proving more useful. Men must be aware that these variations exist so they can make accurate comparisons. Patients must also realize that the increasing number of modifiers of this screening modality attest to its lack of specificity. Lectures at the 2006 AUA Meeting by Dr. D'Amico and colleagues showed that men with a PSAV greater than 1.8 ng/ml per year had a higher incidence of Gleason 7, 8, 9 and 10 tumors.

What are the controversies in using this exam? Some men who have had their prostates removed surgically still have measurable PSA levels. It is thought that this is most likely due to recurrent tumor formation in the post-op site, although many times no cancer is ever found. Researchers from Memorial Sloan Kettering Cancer Center have found that the levels of PSA fluctuate normally and have recommended that an elevated level be repeated. Another study from Harvard and Washington University in St. Louis studied PSA levels in 7,000 men and used mathematical models. Their conclusion was that physicians who waited until the PSA level reached 4 before recommending a biopsy were missing 82 percent of cancer in men under 60 and 65 percent of cancer in men over 60 years of age. The conclusion of the study is that a level of 2.5 should cause consideration of a biopsy. It is well known that biopsy (trauma), infection and benign prostatic enlargement (BPH) can elevate the PSA level. A standard approach has been to place a man with a high PSA on antibiotics for a month. If the number goes down, this implies that the previous increase was due to inflammation.

Dr. Thomas Stamey, Professor of Urology at Stanford University School of Medicine, commenting on the National Cancer Institute's Surveillance, Epidemiology and End Results Program, (SEER), said the program has compiled and released data that show the incidence of death from prostate cancer in men 65 years and older is considerably lower than previously thought. Among men 65 and over, the annual death rate from the disease is 226 per 100,000 population. The article explains, "So, for every 100,000 men over age 65 years old, 40,000 are walking around with invasive prostate cancer—of which only 226 will die annually. The American Cancer Society tells us that close to 40,000 men will die of prostate cancer this year. So, despite all these radical prostatectomies we're doing, we're not making any impact in the death rate."

Dr. Stamey said:

If we were decreasing the death rate, that effect would have become apparent long ago. I think we've been removing too many cancers that are very unlikely to ever bother the patient. Of nine potential morphologic determinants of cancer progression in nearly 400 consecutive cases treated with radical prostatectomy, for every 10 percent increase in Gleason grade 4/5 (Gleason Score 8, 9 or 10), we showed a 10 percent failure rate. He continued by saying, "All the factors we had thought were important, like capsule penetration, seminal vesicle invasion, positive margins, didn't matter."

At the 2004 meeting of the 104th Annual American Roentgen Ray Society, Dr. Catherine Roberts gave a report from the Mayo Clinic that noted men with high grade cancers tended to have low PSA levels. At the same conference, a combined study from the National Institutes of Health in Bethesda and the Stanford University School of Medicine and presented by Dr. J. Alexander highlighted the true nature of the PSA reading. The investigation was made using dynamic contrast enhanced MRI and sophisticated computer analysis which demonstrated elevated levels of PSA were due to vascular permeability (weakness of the blood vessel wall), which could be due to cancer, trauma or inflammation. They were surprised to find patients with low PSA that had cancer and patients with high PSA that had inflammation. This finding was so striking that they called into question other laboratory blood "tumor markers" A report in the April 28, 2004 edition of the *Miami Herald* on new cancer treatments for prostate malignancy cited a 3-D sonogram unit that had high intensity focused ultrasound (HIFU) that killed cancers with minimal damage. This investigation was performed as part of an article of the economics of cancer treatments. The article pointed out that 55 percent of the patients treated by this technique were physicians. It is still true as of this writing that some doctor's accept treatments without the cancer confirmation of the invasive biopsy procedures.

A more even handed view comes from the Prostate Cancer Research Institute's (PCRI) 2004 newsletter. Citing the *New England Journal of Medicine* reports that spurred experts to recommend biopsies at the PSA score of 2.5 ng/ml rather than the current recommendation of 4.0 levels. They noted other professionals disagree, contending that the 4.0 level already results in what they deem to be too many unnecessary biopsies. The PCRI suggests that the issue is more complex than simply changing the threshold and using it as an automatic trigger for giving men biopsies.

The Prostate Cancer Research Institute, *PCRI Newsletters* 2004 and 2005, strongly supports annual testing for the early detection of prostate cancer. Effective testing combines both a PSA blood test and a digital rectal exam for men, beginning at:

- Age 35-for those having a family history of prostate cancer or who are of African/American descent.
- Age 40-for all other men.

The PCRI notes that even elevated PSA levels may indicate the presence of very treatable urinary conditions, such as benign prostatic hyperplasia (BPH) or prostatitis, and do not necessarily indicate that cancer is present in the prostate.

Risk factors, according to the PCRI, are:

- African/American descendents.
- Family history of prostate cancer, especially in brothers.
- High saturated fats and red meat diets.
- Occupations involving pesticides and other chemicals uses.

1. While PSA is a significant indicator in the diagnosis of most forms of PC, there are some extremely aggressive varieties that produce only a small amount of PSA. For this reason PCRI recommends that the DRE as well as the PSA test be done as part of the annual exams.
2. There is a small minority of patients present with disease at an earlier age than indicated by these screening guidelines. Patients are encouraged to research their particular situation and pursue testing PC, if so desired. Any presentation of urinary symptoms (frequency, hesitation, dribbling, pain, incomplete emptying) should be investigated for possible BPH, prostatitis, or PC.

It has been estimated that only 25–35 percent of prostate biopsies each year in the US find PC. Hence, since prostate biopsies involve excising cores of tissue from prostate with needles inserted through the rectum, they should not be performed unless there is a persuasive indication that cancer may be present. However, the presence of a nodule, hardness or irregularity on the DRE is a clear indication for biopsy.

The standard for an elevated PSA has, until recently, been a PSA level of 4.0 ng/ml. However, there is a growing body of research to support that lowering the threshold of the PSA level to 2.5 ng/ml will significantly increase prostate cancer detection. However, it may also increase the proportion of "unnecessary" biopsies.

Prior to taking a PSA test, it should be understood that the PSA test measures an individual's prostate-specific antigen level, and is **not** a prostate-CANCER-specific antigen level. Hence, an elevated PSA level can indicate **prostatitis** (inflamed prostate), **BPH** (non-malignant enlarged prostate), or **prostate cancer.** Both prostatitis and BPH are **conditions**, not diseases that are usually more easily treated, yet whose symptoms may be similar to those of cancer; therefore, a needle biopsy may or may not necessarily be the next reasonable step.

The following should be considered before the decision whether or not to biopsy is made:

1. **Rule out prostatitis.** With the use of a urine culture, antibiotics, and the uPM3 urine test, it may be possible to rule in or rule out prostatitis. If prostatitis is detected, treatment choices should be discussed by the patient and physician.

2. **Rule out BPH.** This can be done (1) by calculating prostate size with the ultrasound measurement of the prostate, (2) by using the uPM3 urine test, and/or (3) with the use of the **free PSA percentage.** The new screening urine test called uPM3 is a genetic test based on a gene made by prostate cancer tissues. This test appears more accurate than the PSA exam.

3. **Rule out high grade cancer that does not make PSA.** Aggressive tumors of high Gleason score may be further evaluated by the following blood tests: **CGA (chromogranin A), NSE (Neuron Specific Enolase), CEA (carcinoembryonic antigen), and PAP (prostatic acid phosphatase).**

Dr. Cornud, the foremost European researcher of prostate color and power Doppler ultrasound has given us a different option. In the journal *Urology* in 1989, he published the following recommendation: If a man has a negative digital rectal exam, a PSA between 4-10 and an unremarkable color or power Doppler sonogram, a biopsy may be deferred. Indeed, in my own practice, many men are choosing this option by themselves.

Discover Magazine, January, 2005 issue notes that the *Journal of Urology* article (October, 2004) reported that the PSA test is currently predictive of cancer in only 2 percent of cases. It also referenced the fact that 80 percent or more of men over age 70 die with—but not from—prostate cancer. The article further quotes Dr. Howard Parnes, an oncologist at the National Cancer Institute saying, "First of all, it is not known how often PSA testing saves lives." The final stinging verdict by both the National Cancer Institute and the American Cancer Society is that the PSA test should be "offered" rather than recommended.

Dr. Robert Getzenberg, director of urologic research at Johns Hopkins University School of Medicine, in the 2007 journal *UROLOGY*, described a new blood test that may replace the PSA as a screening tool. He notes the test is for a protein found only in the nucleus or prostate cancer cells and is called "early prostate cancer antigen-2 or EPCA-2" This is not found in normal cells.

When it enters the blood stream, it remains for a long time and can be measured on a screening basis. Apparently, the levels in the serum can differentiate between organ confined tumor and cancer that has spread beyond the gland. The false positive rate was 3%-meaning no cancer was found when the test indicated a tumor. The false negative percentage was 6%—meaning cancer was found when the test diagnosed no tumor. He noted the specificity of the exam may distinguish between benign disease (BPH and prostatitis) and reduce the estimated 1.3 million to 1.6 million men undergoing yearly biopsies to indentify the 230,000 patients with cancer.

KNOWLEDGE VERSUS PREFERENCE

Merging doctor's knowledge with patient preference is the desired goal in tackling shared decision-making in cancer care. A new model of medical decision-making has emerged that gives patients more responsibility for their own healthcare. The concept of shared decision-making arose in the 1980's. This was partly due from pressures to develop evidence-based strategies for disease prevention and improve treatment outcomes. In cancer care, the idea gained credence with the increasing recognition of two facts:

- Numerous preventive and treatment options involve the potential for significant harm, while holding only limited promise for improvement.
- The fear of the risks and the desire for the benefits of any treatment are highly influenced by patients' personal values and preferences.

Over the years, clinicians have offered patients more information and broader perspective about the risks and benefits of treatments, but many haven't offered patient's true choices that would let them determine for themselves whether or not one option better meets their values or allows them to reject a recommended course of treatment.

As patients and clinicians embrace shared decision-making, particularly between cancer patients, oncologists, or radiation oncologists—patients will play a greater role in determining their treatment plan, including what imaging studies will be performed. Researchers will continue to explore the outcomes of shared decision-making and the value of the tools that clinicians will use to involve patients in their care. "It respects the concept that it's important when making treatment decisions to try to understand and incorporate patients' preferences and information they bring to the decision process," said Tim J. Whelan, BM, BCh, MSc, who moderated a panel discussion on shared decision- making last October at the meeting of the American Society for Therapeutic Radiology and Oncology in Salt Lake City.

Dr. D. Whelan, an Associate Professor in the Department of Medicine and Associate Member of the Department of Clinical Epidemiology and Biostatics at McMaster University in Ontario, Canada, is principal investigator on projects that explore the value of treatment decision aids for women with breast cancer. Decision aids come in many forms, including pamphlets, videos, audiotapes, decision boards, and increasingly, Web-based tools. These aids are not only discussed by the clinician and patient, but they're also typically given to the patient to share and discuss with family, friends, and significant others. For some clinicians shared decision-making provides a way out of the conundrum by giving physicians a method by which they can inform their patients about therapies and procedures that may help some but not others. Doing so allows patients to incorporate their preferences and beliefs into the treatment decision.

TRUE PARTICIPATION

The idea has received numerous labels, including evidence informed patient choice, mutual participation, informed decision-making, and patient-centeredness. There is also ambiguity about the meaning of terms used to describe the interactive decision-making style. For example, some people in medicine believe *informed* decision-making is synonymous with *shared* decision-making. However, the former term merely suggests that patients collect information to better understand their conditions and treatments. It doesn't necessarily imply that patients play a role in choosing their care, nor does it suggest that they solicit the opinions of their doctors.

Similarly, informed consent, which describes the physician's duty to disclose treatment descriptions and to discuss risks, benefits, and alternatives, is not synonymous with shared decision-making. Neither informed consent nor informed decision-making describe the partnership that is at the heart of the newer style of interaction. For many patients, information isn't enough. Shared decision implies two-way information flow between patient and physician that allows them (as a team invested in the patient's best interest) to make medical decisions and plan a clinical course of action. Patients have the information and opportunities with which to articulate their needs, desires, and preferences, and clinicians have the opportunity to express their biases and recommendations.

There's increasing research to indicate that patients want to be better informed," Whelan said, "... but, there's also a wealth of research coming forth indicating that patients want to be involved in decisions about their care; in particular, cancer patients with oncology treatment decisions." Whelan added that there's been growing recognition by clinicians of the importance of incorporating patients' values, preferences, and beliefs in decisions that reflects their wants and desires. "This area of research has been supported by a large body of research documenting unexplained practice variation," said Whelan, "... particularly in areas such as breast cancer surgery, rates of mastectomy, and rates of breast-conserving surgery, but also, in non-oncology areas such as the use of coronary artery bypass surgery."

Many clinicians support such joint decision-making on ethical grounds because it grants patients an autonomous voice and gives them control over their healthcare. On a more practical level, it creates better educated patients, improves patient satisfaction with decisions, increases patient comfort, and builds trust between clinicians and their patients. These advantages, in turn, help reduce the likelihood of malpractice lawsuits.

PHYSICIAN ACCEPTANCE

While many clinicians claim to embrace the concept, fewer rely on it in actual practice for a variety of reasons, including a lack of acceptance by traditional patients who are more comfortable with medicine's usual paternalistic approach. It's also a time-consuming way to treat patients, which can be a daunting challenge in an era of managed care. Curtailed reimbursement forces physicians to see more patients,which pressures them toward spending less time with each patient.

Many clinicians who might welcome the idea, hesitate because of a lack of hard evidence about treatment options. Some are simply not sure how to put the concept into practice or believe they lack the skills to develop true partnerships. The medical literature on the subject has swayed many clinicians to explore the paradigm, but it has not provided overwhelming incentive on a broader scale. Research has not definitively endorsed the shared decision-making concept of patient interaction, but it does suggest that patient satisfaction has increased, and at best, hints at improved outcomes.

There's a wide range of the degree of acceptance by clinicians and an equally broad spectrum of the level of patient participation when their preferences are considered. In some circumstances, shared decision-making is employed through a formal process of established steps; in other cases, it's an informal collaboration between clinician and patient.

BREAST CANCER RESEARCH

It is important to realize that breast and prostate tumors are similar types of cancers. The treatments for breast cancers may be used on the prostate and treatments for prostate cancers may be applied to the breast in many cases. Therefore breast cancer research will ultimately benefit both men and women in future diagnosis and treatment modalities.

Cathy Charles, BA, MA, PhD, Mphil, a medical sociologist at McMaster, who is studying shared treatment decision-making by women with early-stage breast cancer, and the specialists who treat them, spoke about her work to determine how clinicians understand and practice shared decision-making and develop a conceptual framework for the practice of this model. Charles is an Associate Professor in McMaster's Department of Clinical Epidemiology and Biostatistics and an Associate Member in its department of Sociology. She, along with researchers at McMaster, has done conceptual and empirical work in the breast cancer field to determine how radiation oncologists and medical oncologists define shared decision-making, to gauge their comfort level with the concept, and to track the extent to which they actually use the approach in their practice.

In breast cancer treatment risks and benefits necessitate certain tradeoffs. "Outcomes vary in impact on physical and psychological well-being," Charles said, "and in the individual cases, they are uncertain." She traced the evolution of models of decision-making in such cases—from the long-standing paternalistic approach in which information flows in only one direction from physician to patient, to the current, more inclusive attitudes in which information flows in both directions. Among the reasons for the shift, she says, was the recognition that those tradeoffs of quality of life for limited or questionable benefits are subjective—that it's the patients who will have to live or die with the consequences of the treatment decisions and that they ought to have some role in the decision-making process.

POTENTIAL PROBLEMS

Although there is an increasing recognition of the importance of patient input, researchers have also begun to explore problems associated with it. Chief among those concerns is the lack of a clear understanding of the shared decision-making concept. Her group developed a conceptual framework to tease out the meaning of the term and clarify the concept for clinicians. They identified the analytic components of the process—exchanging information, deliberating about treatment options, making the decision on the treatment to implement, and agreeing upon the decision. "We think the framework has practical applications in that it can be used to help evaluate different physician/patient encounters and help in the work of developing decision aids," said Charles. Furthermore, she observed, "It can be used as a tool in professional education to help educate physicians about the different approaches and what steps they might want to take and what skills they would develop in order to use one approach vs. another."

Their research further looked at clinician understanding of the various models of interaction—specifically, shared decision-making, levels of comfort with the latter concept, and the degree to which they use it in practice. Charles noted that their studies revealed a surprisingly high level of consensus about the definition and nature of shared decision-making, about the high degrees of comfort with the idea, but far less about the practical application of the method. "One of our future directions in research," she concluded, "is to further explore why there is this discrepancy between physician comfort level with shared decision-making and the use of this approach." In addition, she said, her group will look at cross-cultural variations as well as patient/physician interaction factors that promote shared decision-making in the oncology encounter.

Whelan, who works with Charles at McMaster, discussed the utility of decision aids and practical dilemmas for clinicians who may wish to use them. "These aids," he explained, "developed as part of an attempt to try to improve patient involvement in decision-making in the clinical encounter to facilitate communication." "Clinicians," he said, "are often faced with weighing potential inconvenience or morbidity caused by adjuvant cancer treatment against the potential reduction in morbidity and mortality later for an individual patient." One reason oncologists struggle with this balancing act is that risks can be high and benefits questionable.

"If we take adjuvant (combination) chemotherapy, benefits may be rather modest, side effects may be truly significant and expected in many cases, and there's still uncertainty," Whelan said. "There's a lack of data for randomized trials, and there's uncertainty about benefits and risks. Even when there are good data from randomized trials," he explains, "and those data are applied from a population basis to an individual—there's still tremendous uncertainty about whether that particular individual will garner a benefit or garner only morbidity from the therapy." "In addition,"he continues," in particular areas of oncology—most notably prostate, breast and colon cancers—there are many options now available to patients."

Whelan suggested that decision aids and shared decision-making will ultimately have an impact in outcomes. "We're at a point now where there is a sufficient number of aids in oncology that oncologists should consider using those that have been developed and shown to be effective in practice," he said. "Our challenge in the clinical encounter is to bridge the gap between knowledge and preferences. We've often thought about that as a clinical art, but we're realizing that science can help us understand that better."

What does the National Cancer Institute caution us about PSA and screening? Below is summarized information publicly available from their website:

There is insufficient evidence to establish whether a decrease in mortality from prostate cancer occurs with screening by digital rectal examination or serum prostate-specific antigen. While some observational studies of men among whom prostate cancer screening was performed have witnessed a fall in prostate cancer mortality, these observations have not been consistent in all populations or within a given population. Furthermore, screening may be accompanied by deterioration in elements of health-related quality of life, primarily due to the complications of therapeutic intervention, e.g., incontinence (both fecal and urinary), urethral stricture, sexual dysfunction, and the morbidity associated with general anesthesia and/or a major surgical procedure.

Although potential harms of screening for prostate cancer can be established, the presence or magnitude of potential benefits cannot; therefore, the net benefit of screening cannot be determined. The prevalence of prostate cancer and precancerous lesions found at autopsy steadily increases for each decade of age, most of these lesions remain clinically undetected. The estimated lifetime risk of the diagnosis of prostate cancer is about 16 percent, and 3 to 4 percent die of this disease. Although DRE has been used for many years, careful evaluation of this modality has yet to take place. Indeed, Thompson's study in the *Scandinavian Journal of Urology*, 1991 reported that 25 percent of men presenting with metastatic disease had a normal prostate examination. The study concluded that the necessity to diagnose or treat a given case of prostate cancer cannot be proven at this time.

The use of androgen deprivation therapy (hormone therapy) or hormone blockage for localized prostate cancer has increased markedly in the last decade. An observational database of 7,195 patients with prostate cancer, including 3,439 men diagnosed since 1989, with clinical staging information available was reviewed. It was observed that patients with clinically localized prostate cancer are increasingly receiving androgen deprivation therapy with radical prostatectomy, radiation therapy, or brachytherapy, although the appropriate role of hormonal therapy in localized disease is unknown. The full impact of increased hormonal therapy on prostate cancer mortality patterns is unknown, according to Cooperberg's article in the *Journal of the National Cancer Institute,* 2003. While there is a consensus about the use of hormone blockade, there is frequently no agreement about the type of blockade to be used or to the optimal duration of treatment. Current studies are trying to clarify this issue, but it will probably take years for this to occur. A logical approach to use for the selection and duration of the hormone treatment is to modulate the intensity of the blockade to the degree of cancer risk. This means stronger treatment for patients with more aggressive disease.

The input of the patient regarding the treatment intensity has little meaning, if the patient doesn't understand the benefits of the particular therapy or the potential side effects. Many of the possible side effects are reversible or preventable with simple measures. For example, osteoporosis (weak bones that fracture), a common side effect may be prevented with a once a week dose of Fosamax or Actonex coupled with weight training. The two other feared complications are loss of libido and energy deterioration.

Libido is a passionate attraction to the opposite sex. This needs to be contrasted with potency, which is the ability to get an erection adequate for vaginal penetration. During hormone blockade, 90 percent of men over age 70 completely lose libido as compared with men under age 50 years who lose libido about 50 percent of the time. Libido returns to normal levels after therapy ceases and testosterone recovers more frequently in younger men. About 50 percent of men over age 70 undergoing two years of treatment never recover testosterone production, which can be supplemented with testosterone gels. Hormone deprivation causes tiredness and weakness especially after 6 months of treatment. The degree varies with each patient and is related to loss of muscle tone and mass and may be counteracted with strength training. Hot flashes are a nuisance, but generally, tolerable. In severe cases progesterone (hormone) shots are helpful. The combination of listlessness and testosterone loss often leads to weight gain, however, dietary adjustments will compensate for this. Breast growth occurs in more that 50 percent of men on anti-androgen hormone therapy which may be treated with radiation therapy or estrogen blocking pills such as Femara. Osteoporosis accelerated bone mass loss occurs in post menopausal women with low estrogen levels and men deprived of testosterone. Untreated this leads to rib, spine and hip fractures (having a 50 percent mortality rate). These side effects may be contained by the modern bisphosphonate treatments such as Fosamax and Actonex pills. Severe cases may require intravenous infusions. Joint pains or arthritis is most common in the hands and may be treated with over the counter preparations such as glucosamine, MSM and Super oxide dismutase (SOD). Standard nonsteroidal anti-inflammatory agents like Motrin and Celebrex are effective remedies.

Memory changes, according to the February, 2005, online edition of *Cancer* include problems with word finding, remembering names and reduction in verbal fluency. Visual recognition and visual memory are also affected. Emotional mood swings occur and may be diminished with common anti-depressant medications such as Zoloft or Paxil. Non cerebral problems include anemia, blood pressure elevation and liver injury. Blood is a mixture of red blood cells and serum (watery fluid). Anemia occurs when the oxygen carrying red cells are depleted resulting in weakness and shortness of breath. Hormone blockade normally drops the blood cell count by 20 percent, which is usually tolerable; however, 10 percent of men develop severe anemia. This is treatable with the hormone erythropoietin or synthetic Aranesp. Blood pressure swings occur both upward and downward and may be adjusted by standard medications. Liver irritation, detected by routine blood tests, may be caused by the commonly used antiandrogens Casodex and Flutamide. Minor injury will lead to severe liver damage if the medicine is not stopped. When the liver function returns to normal, for example, if Casodex was used, Eulexin may be substituted and vice versa.

CHAPTER EIGHT

Assisting the Natural Defense System
of the Body

Studies presented at the May 2005 New York Roentgen Society Annual Meeting in New York showed that imaging with MRI and ultrasound detects cancers better than biopsy alone and should be used to guide biopsies for greater accuracy. Dr. Hedvig Hricak, Director of Radiology at Memorial Sloan Kettering Cancer Center, noted up to 80% of tumors were missed by standard (non image guided) biopsies. In fact, the study also showed that of the successful biopsies, 48% were inaccurately read when compared to the postoperative specimen carefully examined in the pathology department.(The full text of the presentation is appended to the end of the book). Dr. Daniel Kopans, Professor of Radiology at Harvard Medical School, mentioned in his 2005 talk at the New York Cancer Society that current methods were not successful in predicting metastastic potential of cancers and suggested that blood flow analysed by ultrasound Doppler imaging would be helpful. This chapter discusses the time honored nutritional therapies and psychosomatic modalities for controlling cancers. These alternative treatments must be carefully considered given the 11% accuracy of the biopsies, the poor correlation with cancer aggression, the possibility of spreading the malignancy and the 3% overall chance of a tumor being lethal.

A starting point in conquering cancer may be to realize that there is a myth to curing cancer. The above experts have testified to the fact that standard treatments are missing the mark and perhaps there cannot be one "magic bullet" for all patients knowing the wide variety of cancers and the varied response by an individual patient to standardized treatments. Moreover, a cure may prove to be more disabling than the disease itself. Perhaps certain cancers are a natural part of aging and must be dealt with accordingly in a demystified reality. The combination of alternative healing with 21st century progressive medicine offers new hope and realistic choices for cancer victims. The statistics from the beginning of the book show we have not won the fight against prostate cancer. While emergency room medicine is at its pinnacle, re-attaching severed limbs, the same cannot be said of cancer progress. Cancer research funding to extraordinary generous levels have shown we cannot buy a cure for cancer. Searching for a way to live harmoniously with cancer seems a reasonable alternative to finding the elusive cause. Alternative healing provides such an opportunity.

The current treatments of surgery, radiation and chemotherapy have reduced the quality of life for many patients. The side effects of surgery and radiation described earlier, along with the respective 20% and 50% recurrence rate has prompted medical science to seek help from the newer minimally invasive treatments of cryosurgery, RFA and HIFU. Chemotherapy failures have led the chemotherapists to administer ever higher doses of increasingly toxic substances. The nausea and vomiting are often severe enough to require hospitalization. Many patients suffer greatly from the experience. A 2004 report on newer chemotherapies from the New England Journal of Medicine by Dr. Petrylak showed an increase of only 2 months in median survival of men with metastatic prostate cancer. A 2006 study from *BREAST CANCER RESEARCH AND TREATMENT* by Dr. D. Silverman, head of neuronuclear imaging at UCLA School of Medicine, describes the effect of chemotherapy of the brains metabolism noting that patients with "chemo brain" often can't focus, remember things or multitask the way they did before chemotherapy. This effect may last up to 10 years. Newer European protocols combining chemotherapy with other agents that decrease tumor blood flows (thalidomide variations) are showing real promise.

Alternative medicine is coming of age with traditional practitioners who have by now seen first hand the repeated successes of complementary medicine on cancer patients who have sought non conventional treatments elsewhere. Traditionalists have learned that it is best to swim the river in the direction it is going. Taking the best of all healing modalities for a particular patient will prove to be the optimal multidisciplinary approach for the future. When I read the MRI report on a knee in an older patient (degenerative arthritis, torn meniscus, suprapatellar effusion, ACL edema, posterior cruciate tear, tibial cartilage loss, osteophyte formation, cartilage degeneration and internal bone cysts-all in one area) I am surprised that the patient standing in front of me could even walk, much less still play tennis during which activity he had just injured himself. I then ask the patient where he hurts, he points to one area and I show him with the sonogram a partial tear in a ligament that can be healed with physical therapy and rehabilitation. Modern technology looks better at the total disease process than the patient's immediate problem. Todays' physicians look more at the organ (in this case, a knee) and less at the total patient. Much of what is found on MRI or sonograms in the joints is incidental and not clinically significant. I propose we return to treating the patient rather than eradicating the pathology. Medical imaging equipment focuses on disease processes and minimizes the fact that the findings may not fit the clinical situation of the patient's current illness.

In the past, alternative medicine conjured up the vision of back alley treatments in foreign lands. For the last twelve years, I have been following patients with proven cancers who have been successfully treated for their disease. Indeed, some patients who have been told by senior physicians at major medical center to get their affairs in order, come back for follow up scans and are shocked by what I find. They are shocked not at the hopelessness of their situation but rather, by the significant regression of their disease by complementary therapies. I advise my patients to try a treatment that they consider optimal for their lifestyle. We together decide on a follow up visit to come back and see if the therapy is effective and how well it works by using the new scan as an interval comparison with the last 3D PDS study. An example is JW, a college professor, age 43, who came to me a year ago with a "feeling something was wrong in his pelvis." I scanned the prostate with sonogram and found a highly vascular, aggressive region at the base. The MRI confirmed the same findings of a tumor next to, but not involving the seminal vesicle. He wanted to try complementary medicine, but because of his relative youth and the seriousness of the tumor, I advised him to be biopsied at his university hospital. A week and 10 biopsies later, no cancer was found. He went on a complementary treatment as if he had cancer and the blood vessels disappeared 14 days later on a rescan. Six month follow up showed no tumor and he stopped his treatment unilaterally of his own volition without telling anyone. A one year follow up sonogram showed return of the original cancer with spread to both sides and extension out of the prostate. He refuses to have another biopsy and no is no longer a candidate for RFA. He is taking out a loan for his HIFU because he is unwilling to risk losing his potency as he has recently remarried.

Naturopathic healers feel cancer is an outgrowth of a poisoned body and a depleted immune system. A 2005 book by Mitchell Gaynor, MD entitled *NUTURE NATURE NURTURE HEALTH* discusses the environmental impact on health. He cites a class of compounds called "xenoestrogens" which are estrogen mimicking chemicals found in plastics, wood preservers, cleaning solvents, pesticides, herbicides, PCBs used in electric insulators or dioxins and furans that result from burning municipal and toxic wastes. Apparently, more than 3200 chemicals are added to food and the EPA showed that 7.1 billion pounds of 650 industrial chemicals are found in our water and air.

Linking contamination of our food chain with cancer, Dr. Gaynor feels that these estrogen mimicking compounds, which are associated with the onset of breast cancers, are contributing factors in men's prostate cancers. Synthetic hormones (estradiol and progesterone) implanted in cattle to increase their weight produce estradiol levels twenty times higher than normal in some meat products. A similar chemical, bisphenol, appears in many common plastic products-from food wrap to water bottles, and leaches out into liquids we drink. Bisphenol has another dangerous feature, since it is sensed by the body as a chemical hormone similar to those used in clinical hormone therapies, it renders standard hormonal treatments less effective. Lastly, the zinc necessary for optimal prostate health is rendered impotent by metal pollution of lead and cadmium released from burning power plants and hazardous waste incinerators.

Many books have been written on life style alterations and proper nutrition. Men would do well to incorporate these useful ideas into their daily regimens. Nutritious foods are perhaps the easiest and most natural way to protect the body. Nutrient dense fruits and vegetables are more bioavailable than nutrients packaged in pills. This means that the body can utilize the vitamins and minerals and antioxidants more efficiently so they will be more effective in the healing process. Books have been written on the beneficial effects of garlic which may be taken in the form of extracts. In tomatoes, the strong antioxidant lycopene deserves special attention for managing prostate disorders. A 2002 study by Dr. Giovannucci in *Experimental Biology and Medicine* showed that lycopene from tomatoes had a health benefit for prostate cancers, especially the more lethal forms. Therapeutic optimization would include supplemental vitamins, minerals, enzymes and antioxidants for an immune compromised patient. Melatonin, AHCC (active hexose correlated compound), Co-enzyme Q10, olive oil, omega-3 fatty acids have dietary anti oxidant value. Quercitin, resveratrol, ellagic acid, Ip6 (inositol hexaphosphate), TMG (trimethylglycine), selenium, zinc, plant sterols and pomegranate juice are proving valuable as a prostate health supplement. Green tea seems to be the most effective of the tea products.

A clinical trial by Dr. Raymond Oyen, a professor at the medical school in Belgium, was presented at the 2005 JFR meeting. He observed that a plant sterol and antioxidant diet, including vitamin E, soy products and selenium, controlled many patients with precancers (PIN) and true cancers. Recent reports of Co-enzyme Q 10 are showing effectiveness in stabilizing prostate and breast cancers. Cancer researchers,

Drs. Howenstine and Judy, are anecdotally documenting significant tumor regression. Dr. William Judy studied 30 patients with prostate cancer no longer inhibited by hormones and placed them on 500 mg of Co-enzyme Q 10 daily with substantial reduction in PSA levels. At the 2006 Think Tank gathering of international experts under the auspices of the Glaucoma Foundation, it was agreed by many that Co-enzyme Q 10, resveratrol and quercitin combinations helped ward off the dire consequences of the progressive eye disease *glaucoma*.

Parenthetically, the ability of the powerful antioxidants selenium and vitamin E to protect against prostate cancer was found accidentally. In 1996, in a trial to determine whether selenium would influence the rate of skin cancer development, it was found that participants in the study had a 60% lower incidence of prostate cancer. No clinical effect was noted in skin cancer patients.

Likewise, vitamin E, in a 1998 trial, to gauge the preventative effect against lung cancer, showed a 32% decrease in prostate cancer incidence.

SOY PRODUCTS

Although Dr. Oyens' study used soy to prevent cancer development, further study remains essential. It is true that the Japanese eat soy and have lower rates of breast and prostate cancer but they have a higher incidence of stomach cancer. In addition to difficulty in digestion, soy contains protease inhibitors that reduce the efficiency of the digestive pancreatic enzyme trypsin. Dr. Nicholas Gonzalez, a New York City cancer specialist, cautions his patients about eating soy products since he feels pancreatic digestive enzymes are an important anti-cancer entity. Soy beans are high in phytic acid, contained in the hulls of the seed, and block absorption of essential minerals, such as calcium, copper, iron, magnesium and zinc in the intestinal tract. Clearly, soy isoflavone exert hormone effects in the human body, but the overall safety in cancer patients has not been established.

A study of *saw palemetto* by the University of California by Dr. Avins and presented at the 2006 AUA meeting underscored the fact that the extract did not improve flow or urinary symptoms on the standard 160 mg dose twice a day. More troublesome is the understanding that most of this plant comes from Florida in a section that has been designated a toxic waste site. This contamination may explain the increased incidence of hepatitis in patients who take this plant sterol. There may even be a potential use for botulinum neurotoxins (Botox and Myobloc) to paralyse the nerves associated with tumor growth. Anecdotal reports are coming in from breast and prostate cancer patients that neurotoxin injections are clinically stabilizing their tumors with no apparent side effects. Agents such as ozone and light, especially in the ultraviolet wavelength may prove useful in treating disease through the blood system. Books have been written about the Rife energy cancer cure which may yet prove to be a viable resource for patients. Beneficial effect from strong magnetic fields on cancers deserve further evaluation. A book by Dr. John E. Postley, *The Allergy Discovery Diet,* details the devastating effects of food sensitivities leading to allergic reactions which in turn compromise the body's immune system. Dr. Larry Clapp's widely published book on prostate health, *Prostate Health in 90 Days,* has found many avid readers who have changed their lifestyles and improved their prostate disease. Immunotherapies are particularly important for patients who choose surgery, radiation or chemotherapies, since these modalities tend to depress the body's immune system. Studies of *pao periera* and *rauwolfia vomitora* extracts are currently generating clinical interest. An interesting byproduct of the use of herbs, nutritional supplements and dietary changes for treatment of prostate cancer is the accompanying salutary health effects ameliorating heart disease, arthritis, BPH and prostatitis.

Disease, especially cancer is opportunistic. Cancer may be a result of a diseased body debilitated from stress and toxins. Clinical cancer may be a signal from the body that it is out of natural alignment. Westerners for example, do not get parasitic infections when they visit the third world countries at the same rate as the malnourished natives because they have strong immune systems and powerful body defenses stemming from relatively high nutritient diets.

Nutrition is not only food—more important is how your body processes the food you eat. Good nutrition means choosing foods that are naturally rich in valuable nutrients and free from toxic chemicals. It also means eating and drinking foods in such a way that the tissues receive valuable nutrients and not unhealthy byproducts of inadequately digested foods and unhealthy intestinal bacteria. Certified organic foods are free of pesticide residues. Simple and seasonal locally grown products are often helpful. All produce must be washed with a diluted mixture of vinegar or bleach. Grains are highly recommended, however, we must distinguish between processed and whole grains. Also, grains (especially wheat) contain glutens that are a major source of food sensitivity. Most grains and beans contain phytates and enzyme inhibitors that inhibit mineral absorbtion and weaken the intestinal enzymes, often producing flatulence. Vegetables are the core of successful nutrition because they provide phytonutrients, antioxidants, soluble and insoluble fiber as well as essential minerals and vitamins. Equally important is the maintenance of the body acid base balance. Vegetables (and most fruits) prevent the tissues from becoming overly acidic. High cellular acidity prompts the body to use up potassium, calcium and magnesium to buffer or neutralize the acid and realign with the normal slightly alkaline state. High acidity depletes the body of minerals and negatively impacts the immune system. Hyperacidity has been associated with chronic infection, allergies and digestive difficulties.

Avoiding sugar, processed cheese, meat and fried foods will help restore the natural alkaline state of the tissues. Fat is important in the diet since the cell membranes are made from fatty acids. A balance of omega 3/6/9 fatty acids may be obtained by skillful mixing of healthy fats and oils. Specifically, omega 3 and omega 6 compounds regulate inflammation in the body through their transformation into prostaglandins.

The process of digestion is another matter for consideration since food, drink and medicines have different properties affected by the acid environment and mix of good and bad microorganisms in the stomach and intestine. For example, protein breakdown takes much longer than for starch and vegetables. Older patients generate less hydrochloric acid which is essential for protein transformation into amino acids. Men with GERD (acid reflux or gastro-esophageal reflux) have reduced stomach acid due to treatment. Poorly digested food promotes the over-growth of pathologic "bad" bacteria in the small intestine. The acidic and caustic byproducts of indigestion are called "endotoxins" and diffuse out of the intestine into the blood stream and thence throughout the body. Sugar and starch (which converts quickly back to sugar in the gut) provide vital nourishment for the bacteria producing even more internal toxins. Immune system tissues in the bowel and liver may be overloaded, reducing the overall immune response mechanism.

What do antioxidants do? That depends on many factors, so let's review the terms.

- **Antioxidants**
    Molecules that absorb or neutralize free radicals in our cells
- **Carotenoids**
    Yellow, orange and red pigments synthesized by plants which can be converted by the body into vitamin A.
- **Enzymes**
    Proteins found in cells that catalyze biochemical reactions. The most common ones that fight oxidation are Co Q-10 and super-oxide dismutase.
- **Flavonoids**
    Free radical scavenging antioxidants found in many plants.

- **Free Radicals**

   Atoms or molecules possessing unpaired electrons that cause cellular damage.
- **Phytonutrients**

   Term for chemicals in plants including antioxidants.
- **Polyphenols**

   Antioxidant pigments found in many plants.

Antioxidants neutralize free radicals, the oxygen based-based molecules that are a rogue by-product of normal body metabolism. Most commonly found in DNA, cell walls and interiors, free radical molecules differ from normal molecules in one significant respect: they contain an odd or unbalanced number of electrons. Normal, stable molecules have an even number of paired electrons, whereas, in free radicals, one electron is missing its partner. This imbalance makes the molecule highly unstable so it searches for another single electron and steals it from another normal molecule. The theft of an electron turns this molecule into a free radical which sets up a cascade of electronic theft producing oxidative damage or oxidative stress.

There are two ways antioxidants disrupt this process:
1. Some substances break the chain reaction, decreasing the production of free radicals
2. Others donate electrons to the scavenging molecules returning them to a stable state

Free radicals produce oxidative damage to the DNA causing mutations. They produce oxidative stress to the lipids that make up the cell walls reducing their protective functionality. Our body has its own antioxidant cleanup system rendering free radicals harmless. The following dramatically increase the body's free radical level:
- Sun exposure
- Smoking
- Excess alcohol consumption
- Excess caffeine consumption
- Chronic stress
- Overeating-the more food metabolized, the more free radicals formed
- Undereating-quick weight loss diets burn fat more quickly releasing free radicals

While there exist thousands of known antioxidants, experts believe than hundreds of thousands may be eventually discovered. Antioxidants come in animal, mineral and botanical sources. Animal cells (humans, fish, livestock) manufacture the important enzymes Co Q-10, glutathione and super-oxide dismutase. These act by fighting free radicals and catalyzing chemical reactions that stabilize the free radicals. Our body makes these substances, however, disease states require greater amounts for combating pathogens, so a natural fermented form is often used. There is a synthetic variety currently available which is not well absorbed by the body. Mineral sources include zinc, copper and selenium. These must be carefully balanced since overdosage of any one mineral may be harmful. Botanical sources are the vast majority of chemical defenses against free radicals. Vitamins A, C and E are especially useful. Vitamin A works by quenching free radicals. Vitamin C offers up free electrons to the molecules that crave them. Vitamin E prevents oxidation by breaking the free radical chain reaction.

Thousands more botanical antioxidants are called phytonutrients and fall into three categories;
1. Flavonoids, a group that currently includes more than 4,000 chemicals, are all purpose scavengers because they find free radicals and then neutralize them by donating electrons. Quercitin, found in vegetables, dark cholcolate and fruit skins, is especially active in this function. A large subcategory is polyphenols and phenolic compounds found in grapes, blueberries, pomegranates, cherries, raspberries, cranberries, grains and black and green tea; Resveratrol occurs in minute quantities in redwine.
2. Lignans: from seeds, like flax and sunflower.
3. Carotenoids: found in tomatoes, carots, watermelon and spinach. The two main antioxidants are lycopene and lutein.

A rationale for holistic regimens to combat cancers come from the 2007 American Society of Clinical Oncology presentation of Dr. De Marzo, a pathologist at Johns Hopkins, and Dr. Nakai, of Osaka University in Japan entitled *Inflammation and Prostate Carcinogenesis.* Twenty percent of malignancy comes from chronic oxidative inflammatory states usually provoked by a combination of infectious agents and environmental exposure. Chemoprevention, better known as alternative medicine, is the use of agents preventing the induction, growth or progression of tumors. PIN or *prostatic intraepithelial neoplasia* seems to be a precursor for invasive prostate cancer and is detected only by biopsy. The standard medical treatment for this condition is to watch and wait. Antioxidant treatments block the inflammatory LOX (lipoxygenase) enzymes and may help prevent PIN from progressing to aggressive cancer. The relationship between antioxidant pathways and highly aggressive "interval cancers" is undergoing intensive study at this time.

Malignant cell mutations occur within the body tissues continually and are regularly extinguished or inactivated by the body's defense mechanisms. Cancer cells are held in check by the immune system, which is the body's natural defense system. The immune system is made up of organs (like the skin and stomach) and cells (like white blood cells) that protect the body from dangerous agents. Lymphocytes (white blood cells) that kill cancers are called B cells, NK (natural killer) cells and T cells. These defensive cells attach themselves and kill anything foreign to the body. Other cells remove the inactivated cancer cells and the liver, kidney, lungs and digestive system ultimately discharge them from the body.

Complementary medicine seeks to treat the underlying cause that disabled the body's natural defenses and allowed the tumor to grow. While immune system dysfunction sets the stage for cancer growth, it is the stress to the immune system that incapacitates this vital force from successfully attacking and disabling newly formed tumor cells. The stress comes in the form of damaging free radicals that destabilize normal cells. Common physical stress items include high fat diets, alcohol, food additives, smoking and radiation. Psychological stress and depression take a high toll of the immune system by depleting the will to live. Most physicians understand that there is a connection between disease of the body and emotional imbalances in the mind.

Psychotherapy is useful for some, however, laughter, music, and strong commitments seem to be more beneficial to improve general psychological health. Art therapy and occupational therapy have been applied successfully to mental problems for years. Yoga, martial arts such as Tai Chi and aerobic exercise are standard relaxation protocols in today's high stress world. Meditation has lowered blood pressure and improved lives for half a century in America. Studies have shown where there is hope, there is life. Patients, under anesthesia for cancer surgery, who over hear the operating room staff discuss the full extent of a bad tumor and the hopeless of the patients condition, die much sooner than expected by the natural course of the disease process. Even the unconscious mind affects our health. Patients who fight for life live longer. Patients who give up the fight to live often die prematurely.

In my medical career of nearly half a century, I have investigated the reasons for people living in spite of being pronounced dead at university hospital emergency departments. Simply put, they refused to die even though their physical body appeared dead to our sophisticated diagnostic instruments and highly trained emergency department physicians. This was especially true of the US Air Force pilots I treated during the Vietnam conflict who had sustained massive trauma and survived when they had no medically reasonable chance of pulling through. A lady friend, an avid cyclist, was struck by a car in lower Manhattan 15 years ago. She was brought to the ED at Bellevue Hospital Center, considered the best trauma facility in the Northeast United States. She was pronounced dead. He pupils were fixed and dilated. She heard the doctors calling the time of her death out loud. She felt the large IV pulled out of her arm. She kept saying to herself, "I'm not going to die. I'M NOT GOING TO DIE!" She opened her eyes and coughed. The sheet was pulled away from her face. The IV was reinserted. She lived. After 6 months of rehabilitation, she was told she could never swim due to the surgical scarring under both arms. Yes, she now swims. She has become a sought after public speaker on what is possible in life. Perhaps the will to live is nature's strongest antioxidant. Conversely, there is the entity called "voodoo death." In an attempt not to give a cancer patient false hope, a physician may tell a patient he has 6 months or a year to live. An article by Dr. Cannon in 2002 *American Journal of Public Health* referred to this emotional guillotine that disconnects the patients will to live by severing his lifeline with possibility based on his physician's "sentence" of probable reality. Cancer surviors are not statistics, they are people with courage and the overriding will to live. It is your choice to be the exception rather than the example.

I can attest to the fact that cancer support groups have great psychological value. When I lecture for these groups, I am encouraged to hear so many prostate cancer survivors proclaim that their post cancer life is better and more meaningful that their pre-cancer existence. Not only do many men feel better and function at a higher physical level than before they were diagnosed with their malignancy, but they enjoy life more. In fact, their body is often in better physical shape due to a dynamic change of life style and their satisfaction level is usually higher due to a new appreciation of life. Prayer is frequently a source of peace of mind that translates into a healthful and more positive future.

Finally, patients must have hope in the future of medicine to find new modalities for treating cancer. The non invasive and minimally invasive therapies I have discussed in this book were not in the thoughts of most specialists in the cancer field. My foundation, the Biofoundation for Angiogenesis Research and Development, is continually searching the frontiers of medical science to extract, document, refine and ultimately bring to patients the myriad of new possibilities for treating malignancies. Incorporating successful therapies for other diseases into prostate treatments may be useful, since there are known similarities between breast cancer and prostate malignancies. An article by Lawrence Altman, MD, medical editor of *The New York*

Times, in the May 15th 2005 edition noted that a drug used to treat breast cancer may be prevent men with precancerous prostate conditions from developing full blown malignancy. Dr. Altman cited findings from the annual meeting of the American Society of Clinical Oncology. Men with the condition "prostate intraepithelial neoplasia," or P.I.N., for short, tend to develop malignant tumors over time, somewhat like colon polyps often turning cancerous. The drug, toremifene, blocks the action of estrogen hormone, and has proved useful in preventing breast cancer. The men with PIN developed prostate cancer 1/3 less often than those without the medication in the trial group. While it is widely accepted that the hormone testosterone fuels prostate cancer, there is now evidence that the female hormone estrogen may also stimulate some prostate malignancies. The clinical trial was designed to treat prostate cancer with fewer hormonal side effects. The article also cited other non cancer treating agents that are showing cancercidal effects in certain tumors to the surprise of the medical community.

Another author postulating possible anti-cancer effects from a commonly used drug, botulinum neurotoxin-A (Botox) is Dr. Antonella Giannantoni, MD, Ph.D, a urologist at the University of Perugia Medical Center in Italy. In material presented at the 2005 International BPH Forum in San Antonio, Texas, it seems that injections of this toxin may slow down cancer cell mitosis (division and growth). Animal studies over the years have also shown cell death attributed to neurotoxin. A multicenter study by Drs. Chancellor from the University of Pittsburg Medical School and Chuang from Taiwan presented at the 2005 International Continence Society in Montreal also showed the neurotoxin effects in the rat prostate included decreased activity and cell death within two weeks. Dr. Gallez, a professor of pharmacy from Belgium, has observed the neurotoxin to potentiate cell death from radiation and chemotherapy according to a 2006 study published in *Clinical Cancer Research.* The sister drug, botulinum neurotoxin-B (Myobloc) is also being studied for this effect.

Clearly, an open mind to any and all therapies, combined with well designed clinical trials, will further advance cancer survival and improve quality of life for cancer patients. This is illustrated by a presentation at the 98th Annual Meeting of the 2003 American Urologic Association in Chicago by a Dr. Miroslav Zalesky, a urologist from Prague, Czechoslovakia. He noted that blood vessels observed by the 3D PDS technology in the prostate determined extracapsular spread with 89% accuracy in a series of 282 patients. The spread of abnormal vessels from the gland through the capsule was highly significant and best demonstrated using the 3D capability for interpretation. Dr. Zalesky felt that 3D reconstruction enables physicians to biopsy areas of suspicious neovascularization (new abnormal arteries and veins) that would be missed by the standard sextant biopsy. In a commentary on this study, Dr. Michael Brawer, a urologist not involved in the study, and quoted in the April 30th 2003 issue of *Doctor's Guide* on the internet, said: "it is uncertain at this point whether the new modality can detect the fine vessels that are typical of the neovascularization found in cancer." "The problem is that the size of the vessel delineated with Doppler is larger than the vessels found in malignancies," said Dr. Brawer. "Are our imaging modalities sensitive enough to identify the small vessels characteristic of cancer? I don't know." While Dr. Brawer may be correct, he may also be missing the point that we do not need to see the small vessels associated with cancer to identify tumors. This reminds me of the story of a friend who borrowed my new car years ago in the summertime and reported back that the air conditioning was broken. It worked better on low than on high speed. She was right, and also missed the point since the AC was functioning perfectly well, but her understanding of its operational principles was not. In the New York City traffic, the motor did not revolve quickly enough at slow speed to make the air conditioner system run efficiently, hence it did not work on the high setting. On the open highway, at optimal driving conditions, the AC cooled the car adequately at the lowest setting, so a higher setting was not tried. Physicians need a cancer marker that works, rather than an indicator that fit's their current expectations. To paraphrase Galileo, if a fact is verifiable and pertinent, it does not matter if it makes sense or dovetails with our "gold standard" academic paradigms. No matter how inconceivable, a true discovery must be fully investigated. Imagine if Sir Isaac Newton had thought the wind caused apples to fall. Just as alternative treatments need a chance to be verified, so do anecdotal observations that fall outside of today's traditional medical values.

A remedy proposed and validated by Dr. Majid Ali, Board Certified Surgeon and Board Certified Pathologist, is that of "dysoxygenosis and oxystatic therapy." In his 2004 book *Principles and Practice of Integrative Medicine*, Dr. Ali shows a lack of oxygen to cause disease states and demonstrates successful therapies that re-oxygenate the body emphasizing the use of hydrogen peroxide, ozone, oxygen and related substances that promote healing.

CHAPTER NINE
Emerging Scientific Discoveries

THE PROSTATE CAPSULE

Much emphasis has been placed by patients and physicians on extension of cancer outside the fibrous covering of the prostate gland. This so called extracapsular extension (ECE) was supposed to mean the cancer is inoperable and presumably fatal in the long term. Noted earlier in the book, pathology studies have shown that MRI depiction of this entity is at best 90% accurate. More important, clinically localized cancers are proven to lie outside the prostate at least 50% of the time. Dr. Stylianos Lomvardias, a urologic pathologist, formerly at the AFIP (Armed Forces Institute of Pathology) has described normal prostate glands in the muscle outside the prostate borders. Surgeons often find the capsule difficult to visualize during the operation. Perhaps the focus of treatment should be the location of the cancer in or out of the prostate gland and the invasiveness as demonstrated by PDS rather than the "sentence" of inoperability when it has spread beyond the elusive capsular wall. Dr. Robert O'Connor, a urologic pathologist from the University Hospital in Ireland, has also attested to the fact that the so called capsule is often difficult to demonstrate in the post-operative specimen.

Two major presentations at the 2007 AUA meeting discussed the accuracy of imaging the prostatic capsule. A multicenter study from Harvard and the Medical College of Georgia looked at EC-MRI (endorectal probe coil) in determining pre-operatively the status of the prostate capsule. Sixty two patients had radical prostatectomies with special attention to ECE (extracapsular extension) 80% of T1C (clinically localized) cancers had positive margins at the operative pathologic review. The conclusion was EC-MRI was not valid in assessing ECE in prostate cancer. A larger study from the Medical University Insbruck of 180 patients using 3D-PDS showed 84% sensitivity, 96% specificity and an overall accuracy of 92% in detecting ECE. Furthermore, the positive predictive value (number of expected ECE cases) was 94% and the negative predictive value (number of expected non-ECE margins) was 91%. Of greatest interest was the 90% accuracy in detecting seminal vesicle invasion. Their conclusion was the 3D PDS was an accurate technique for staging localized prostate cancer, and, in the case of advanced disease, the detection of capsular perforation and seminal vesicle invasion was high.

CONTRAST ENHANCED DOPPLER SONOGRAPHY

The ability to better image blood vessels by injecting an enhancing agent intravenously has been used in Europe and Japan for several years. This is not FDA approved in the United States as of this writing. Drs. F. Frauscher and G. Bartsch, in their 2006 presentation at the 92nd Scientific Assembly of the Radiologic Society of North America noted that this simple technique improved vessel detection allowing for targeting these areas and finding more cancers. In 3446 patients screened with this modality, the overall cancer detection rate was 32%. However, one third of tumors occurred in men with a PSA between 2.0–3.9 ng/ml and these were men in the lower age groups.

Another use of this technology is to predict treatment outcome. Dr. Y. Kono, in the 2007 *Journal of Vascular and Interventional Radiology* found blood flow regression to occur as early as two (2) days after successful intraarterial chemotherapy. These treatment results are normally available after three (3) months by standard CT and MRI exams. While this work was performed on liver cancers, it portends well for predicting therapeutic outcome for any vascular tumor. This minimally invasive modality may reduce the need for biopsy sampling to ensure a clinically effective endpoint. A 2007 article in *Journal of Urology* by Drs. Mitterberger and colleagues from the Medical University of Innsbruck, Austria showed that contrast enhanced color Doppler biopsies showed higher grade tumors better than routine biopsies. While this contrast agent has been denied approval by the FDA, it appears that the latest generation of power Doppler units which became available in the United States early 2007 will prove an accurate substitute for this minimally invasive intravenous technology.

SONO-ELASTOGRAPHY

European and Japanese investigators have developed a novel way to show the toughness of tissue using special ultrasound properties showing the elasticity of investigated organs. Cancer tissue is usually firmer than benign tumorous tissue which is, in turn, harder than normal tissue. When I place a needle to biopsy a cancer, I can feel the gritty nature of the malignant area during the aspiration or biopsy process. A needle inside a benign lesion often has a rubbery, softer feel. Normal tissues tend to have little resistance to the needle passage. Palpation to assess a tumor has been part of medicine since Hippocrates. The measurable quality of firmness in diseased tissue was studied over 200 years ago by a British physician, Thomas Young, and is related to the deformation of an area when subjected to physical stress forces. Elastography is comparable to using computers instead of fingers to examine abnormal areas using the basic principles first articulated by Dr. Young.

Elastography, using sonographic equipment and special computer analysis, was perfected by the Laboratory of Waves and Sound in Paris and has been performed in breast cancer diagnosis for several years with significant success. Equipment developed by the Curie Institute in Paris is being used to measure the severity of liver cirrhosis (scarring) and healing in response to medical treatment. This has been so accurate, that this has replaced liver biopsies to ensure improvement has occurred. Drs. L. Pallwein and F. Frauscher in their 2006 Radiologic Society of North America oral presentation and paper in the 2007 *Current Opinons in Urology* observed this was a useful but as yet not highly specific diagnostic test. In breast cancer studies, a negative test is being used to defer biopsies in some patients. European studies are showing that sonoelastography guided biopsies target the cancer 2.8 times more accurately than without this technology. A 2007 article in *Journal de Radiologie* by Dr. Anne Tardivon from the Curie Institute showed a 96.7% negative predictive value in breast tumors, meaning that minimally suspicious tumors could be watched rather than biopsied. This technique may eventually used to stage the spread of cancer. Drs. Pallwein and Frauscher, who use the same ultrasound unit I have, reported in the 2007 ECR meeting many false positives (275 out of 533 suspicious areas) yet feel it is truly valuable as more experienced is gained. However, the stiffness of the seminal vesicles by cancer infiltration and tumor penetration through the capsule had higher accuracy when compared with MRI findings. Their article in 2007 *British Journal of Urology* noted false positives in the presence of stones, chronic prostatitis and tumors smaller than 5 mm. Many ultrasound equipment manufacturers are currently developing a more sophisticated versions specific for the prostate. These will be simultaneously tested in international venues and the results will be presented in the next edition of *PROSTATE CANCER DECODED*.

To add to the innovative combinations of diagnostic testing, engineers, physicists and radiologists have now merged elastography with RFA. Drs. Lee and Varghese in the 2003 *American Journal of Radiology* have used sono-elastography to confirm that thermal treatments have been effective. The article showed the 3-D elastographic images correlated very well with the pathologic specimen of the treated tissues. This now provides another parameter for therapeutic progress that is essentially instantaneous and avoids the need to verify success by CT or MRI scans days later. The success of the procedure will be assessed immediately following treatment and additional ablation may be performed in a timely manner. Dr. Konig in 2005 *Journal of Urology* used elastography to guide prostate biopsies in a series of 404 patients and demonstrated an 84% success rate. This two year study used the same 3D PDS unit that I have had for 4 years, however the power Doppler function was not compared with the elastography feature.

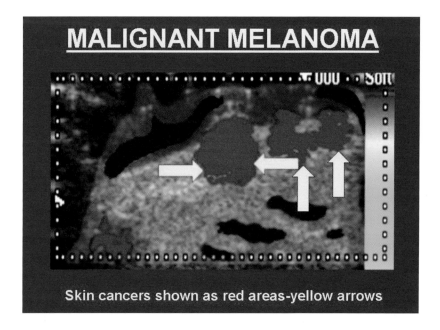

Figure 9.1 Skin cancers (red areas) are harder than benign tumors

3 TESLA MRI (3T-MRI)

The usual MRI scan employs a magnet using a magnetic field strength of 1.5 Tesla. In the past few years higher magnetic field strengths have become available, so 3.0 Tesla systems are now being utilized. The higher field strength shortens the exam time so fewer minutes are spent inside the magnet tube-a blessing for the claustrophobic. While some increase is resolution is usually obtained, the systems are not yet fully optimized as of this writing for examining the prostate. Unfortunately, tiny pieces of metal in the eye or other parts of the body that would not be affected by a 1.5 Tesla magnet, may be pulled towards a higher field strength system, possibly resulting in injury to the patient and conceivably causing blindness. 7 Tesla units are currently being tested on animal prostates with impressive results.

COMPUTER AIDED FULL TIME POINT DCE (CONTRAST ENHANCED)-MRI

During the past four years paramagnetic gadolinium contrast has been injected intravenously to highlight cancer detection during the MRI examination. This is called contrast enhanced (CE) or dynamic MRI sequencing. While this had improved visualization of tumors, computer aided detection has been more advantageous in determining tumor aggression. Developed by an Israeli scientist, Hadassa Degani, PhD, we have been using the process in breast and prostate cancer patients for two years. Contrast flows into the venous system and diffuses into and out of the prostate. This is called the wash-in and wash-out principle. Abnormal wash-in/wash-out occurs in cancers due to the abnormal vessel caliber and increased vascularity which results in vascular permeability (leaky vessels) and detectable contrast in the tumor space. The computer program color codes the cancer red and the normal tissue blue. This is quantifiable and used as a baseline for treatment as is demonstrated in the cover of the book. This is especially important in patient care since the effect of chemotherapy may be demonstrated in some breast cancers within a few days following the first treatment. We have been following up high grade prostate cancers within 3–7 weeks of treatment with 3D PDS and FTP-MRI and seen dramatic reversal of hypervascularity in most cases. If a therapeutic result is not achieved within 12 weeks in the prostate tumor, consideration is given to other medical management. Breast and prostatic cancers are often multifocal and may be of different degrees of aggression. Sequential 3D PDS and FTP MRI are optimizing treatment decisions. Clinicians are beginning to favor this accurate color coded imaging modality over the S-MRI technologies since we are able to detect the small tumors routinely missed by current spectroscopic protocols. Perhaps the addition of 3 Tesla magnets will improve the specificity of S-MRI. In our practice, the addition of FTP MRI has permitted the avoidance of the ER coil which is both time consuming and uncomfortable. Remember that prolonged exam time results in more patient motion and ER coil motion often occurs without injections to paralyze the colon. Motion artifact is devastating to MRI images and the FTP MRI system has decreased motion by improving patient comfort thereby improving imaging resolution. Aside from the added cost of the ER coil MRI, most patients refuse to have the process repeated due to the often painful insertion process. Colorized FTP MRI images are usually available within an hour or two of the scan sequence. In similar manner to the 3D PDS imaging, blood flow parameters of MRI are being studied and proving clinically effective. At our center, we are using the proven 3D Doppler technology to calibrate the newer computer aided MRI flow sequences. As the FTP MRI is improved, new secrets of blood flow within cancers may be revealed so that the 3D PDS imaging may also be improved. Contrast agents for the prostate are not currently approved by the FDA in the United States. Technologies currently on the horizon include MRI particles that can bring chemotherapeutics directly to the tumorous region sparing normal tissues.

LYMPH NODE MRI (LNMRI)

Part of the reason for treatment failures with pelvic cancers is the presence of small nodes and hidden nodes that cannot be visually identified by the surgeon. Some or all of these may contain cancerous cells. Drs. Harisinghani and Saksena presented three papers at the ARRS 2007 meeting demonstrating the new technique of MRI imaging lymph nodes distinguished between unremarkable glands and cancer filled nodes. Under MRI guidance, abnormal findings were biopsied. This means that unsuspected cancer spread may be discovered and treatment appropriately altered. 3.7% of patients in the study were shown to have perirectal nodes (invisible glands around rectum) that were small to medium pea sized (4–8 mm). Perirectal nodes are not evaluated during routine surgical removal of the lymph node chains making MRI and/or 3D ultrasound imaging with a special unit designed to evaluate the perirectal space the modality of choice to ensure full diagnostic accuracy. Our foundation's ongoing study with the Dutch Cancer Center in Nijmegen, Netherlands is fortunately demonstrating that not all the abnormal nodes detected by MRI are cancerous. The results of this investigation will be reported in the next edition of this book.

POSITRON EMMISON TOMOGRAPHY—PET SCANS

In earlier chapters, PET scan technology available in the United States was in the limited value category for prostate evaluation, even though it is being widely used for other cancer detection. European advances by Dr. Jean-Noel Talbot in Paris are permitting diagnostic use of this modality within the prostate as noted in the 2006 *American Journal of Radiology*. PET is a radioactive substance that is injected into the vein and localizes in abnormal tissues. Since this is excreted by the kidneys, it fills the bladder and obscures the prostate. More importantly, many prostate cancers and their metastatic sites grow more slowly than most other more aggressive cancers and have a lower uptake of the glucose based isotope resulting in decreased sensitivity. CT imaging produces an overlay providing anatomic triangulation of the diseased organs. This used glucose (sugar) based isotope and is called FDG PET scan. Outside the US, a PET radioactive isotope using *choline* instead of glucose is called FCH PET or choline-PET scan. Remember, spectroscopic MRI uses choline as a metabolic marker. Technicalities aside, the resolution of this scan greatly improves detection of the cancer within the prostate and better localizes the spread of the disease.

PROSTATE SIZE REDUCTION BEFORE DEFINITIVE CANCER TREATMENT

It is intuitively obvious that the smaller the prostate gland the better the effectiveness of the cancer treatments. The Europeans who employ the HIFU Ablation technology first reduce the size of the gland by surgically removing the benign enlargement by TURP (trans urethral resection prostate) before beginning HIFU treatment. They have shown the smaller the gland the shorter the treatment. Also the chance of urinary obstruction is lessened because the postoperative gland swelling produces less impingement on the urethra. This shortens the recovery time as well. Over 1000 cases have been successfully performed with this pretreatment size diminution. HIFU is optimally performed in glands under 50 cc in size. One unfortunate side effect presented at the 100th Annual AUA Meeting in 2005 was that the TURP procedure had a high association with painful ejaculations after men had this surgery. Radiation and hormone therapies are also used to shrink the prostate volume prior to certain treatments.

These methods have significant side effects detailed earlier in the book. A new technique is emerging as a less traumatic modality to offer the benefits of a smaller prostate for definitive cancer treatments. In 2000, researchers from the Department of Surgery at the Catholic University Hospital in Rome began injecting the deadly poison *botulinum neurotoxin* type a into the prostate to improve symptoms of benign enlargement. During the course of a year, prostate volume decreased by half and symptoms improved. This was performed by manual injection without ultrasound guidance. No significant side effects were reported. Thereafter, studies by the Mayo Clinic using ultrasound guided injections of Botox and the University of Perugia Medical Center in Italy also using ultrasound guidance were performed. Presented at the 2005 American Urological Association Meeting, before 10,000 urologists, was the statement by Dr. Thayne Larson of the Mayo Clinic that the injcction was harmless and "Botulinum Toxin has the potential of being an important change in the way we treat LUTS (lower urinary tract symptoms) in the office."

The next paper at the meeting was by Drs. Guercini, Giannantoni and me citing our work separate from the Mayo Clinic study and verifying the safety and the sometimes remarkable reduction in prostate volume of this procedure. Indeed, one of our patients from England dramatically reduced his gland size from 130 to 40 cc (6x normal to 2x normal) in just a month. This observation prompts the question: could injection of *botulinum neurotoxin* be a way to reduce the size of an enlarged prostate gland prior to HIFU, surgery or radiation. Our group has begun an investigation to compare *botulinum neurotoxin a (Botox)* and *botulinum neurotoxin b (Myobloc)* to see if there is a significant difference between the two pharmaceuticals. The ultimate intent is to use both these commercially available preparations to rapidly reduce the size of the prostate so that cancer treatments will be more rapidly available. It currently takes 3–6 months before hormone treatments reduce the size significantly. In the case of a man with a high grade cancer and a 60 cc prostate, the injection shortening the time from 6 months to one month would prove miraculous. The use of ultrasound guidance permits injections to avoid the site of the cancer and decrease the risk of cancer cells spreading outside the prostate while delivering a therapeutic dose to the site of the benign enlargement. The 3-D/4-D ultrasound probe allows the most accurate positioning of the needle. Since needle placement is optimized, we are able to use a small (22 gauge) needle that is virtually painless during the insertion and injection phases. It is our hope this pretreatment method will make the following minimally invasive treatment procedures more effective.

A new drug Avodart (dutasteride) follows a similar chemical pathway as Proscar (finasteride) and is proving helpful in shrinking the prostate with few side effects. Long term problems have not been studied so the overall safety of dutasteride cannot be guaranteed at this time. Antioxidant therapies are likewise proving effective in diminishing prostate size. One patient with a 900 cc (think *grapefruit*) prostate shrunk the gland down to 300 cc within 8 months and has maintained the size between 250 to 340 cc for the last two years with this regimen. He claims the only trouble he has urinating is when he becomes constipated.

RADIOFREQUENCY ABLATION AND THERMOTHERAPIES

Dr. Bruno Fornage, an Interventional Radiologist at the MD Anderson Cancer Center in Texas, has studied radiofrequency ablation (RFA) outside the usual guidelines. While this technique has been successfully applied to tumors of the liver, kidney, lung, brain, and (in Europe) the prostate, Dr. Fornage studied small tumors of the breast and published his findings in the 2004 *Radiology*. Twenty-one patients with malignancies were treated with RFA prior to surgical mastectomy. The results of examining the specimens showed that this technique is both feasible and safe in tumors less than 2 cm in size. In Belgium, Drs. Zlotta, from the Erasme Hospital in Brussels and Dr. Michael Marberger, a Professor of Urology from Vienna, treated 15 patients with prostate cancer using RFA. Their published results in the *British Journal of Radiology*, 1998 show the destruction of the cancers was reproducible and controlled. While small tumors of the prostate may be treated with RFA with few side effects, it is a challenge to consider treatment of the entire gland due to the adjacent structures of the rectum, nerves and bladder. Hopefully, the advances made in cryosurgery and HIFU may be applied to this evolving technology. Isolating the prostate gland from the rectum and bladder by the use of saline injection to form a protective liquid shield may allow the more aggressive use of larger needles to treat the entire prostate and surroundings with acceptable complication rates.

Drs. Neeman and Wood from the Diagnostic Radiology Department of the National Institutes of Health Clinical Center and the National Cancer Institute, published an article for *Techniques in Vascular and Interventional Radiology* 2002 discussing newer uses of RFA. Noting a complication rate less than 3 percent for the over 3,000 treatments of liver cancer, the authors felt that destroying tumors by de-bulking (surgically making the cancer smaller to improve the quality of life) is a technique showing much promise. Several companies make this equipment. Each of the units has advantages and disadvantages. Of vital importance is the patient selection for this procedure. Patients with small and isolated tumors that are distant from major blood vessels, bowel, nerves and bladder make the best candidates.

This is a team procedure and consultation with surgical oncologists, pain control specialists and palliative care practitioners is useful in pre-procedure evaluation. For small and localized areas, local or intravenous anesthesia is useful, while for larger invasive regions, spinal or general anesthesia may be used. A post-op patient controlled analgesia pump may be administered for large treatment sites. The 3-D sonographic imaging accurately allows placement of the metallic tines of the radiofrequency antennae in position, and the procedure may be completed in about 20 minutes for a 1 cm tumor. Vascular tumors successfully treated no longer show blood flows upon termination of the heating. A useful feature of this modality is that the entry path for the treatment needle may be cauterized upon exiting to destroy any malignant cells seeded in to the needle site. This access tract heating also controls bleeding. One expected complication in the prostate would be swelling of the prostate that would prevent urination. This can be treated prophylactically with an indwelling penile catheter or a suprapubic (bladder) catheter, which may be more comfortable. However, small tumors away from the urethra may not cause urinary obstruction, so that the patient could be monitored for voiding difficulties in this situation. An animal study from Boston's Dana Farber Cancer Institute and the Harvard Medical School authored by Dr. Nahum Goldberg on a method of improving RFA appeared in *RADIOLOGY* May 2005. The article noted better tissue destruction if RFA was combined with intravenous chemotherapies. Hopefully, this synergistic effect will prove useful in humans in the near future.

CANCER INDUCED ANGIOGENESIS AND ANTIANGIOGENETIC DRUGS

Angiogenesis (from the Latin: angio=blood vessel, genesis=creat) or new blood vessel formation in tumors, plays a pivoted role in the development and progression of cancer. The high prevalence of cancer induced growth of arteries and veins makes these vessels a logical target for cancer therapy. Antiangiogenesis therapy, that is, treatment to destroy the blood vessels supplying a tumor, has several theoretical advantages. First, the tumor blood vessels are generally more homogeneous than the tumor cells. Secondly, the lining cells of the vessels are stable so acquired drug resistance may be rare. Third, a partial damage to the lining cells may be enough to block blood supply to a tumor resulting in growth inhibition or even shrinkage of the cancer. This treatment requires imaging the arteries and documenting changes in the blood vessels and its effect on the tumor. The importance of angiogenesis was best stated at the JFR2006 in Paris by Professor N. Grenier: *la neoangiogenese precede les etapes significatives de croissance tumorale:* translated: the tumor growth depends on the presence of new blood vessels.

The ability to demonstrate these vessels will not only improve diagnosis, but will further research and development of newer treatments.

What is the optimal test to look at arteries? The following are criteria for an ideal vascular imaging technique:

- Non-invasive
- Risk free
- Completed in less than 60 minutes
- No expensive monitoring required-no nursing or post procedure recovery expense
- Free of ionizing radiation

- No danger to the kidneys-no dye (iodinated contrast) utilization
- Painless
- Applicable to all patients
- Objectively and easily performed
- Easy to interpret by trained personnel
- Cost effective
- Provide 3-D rendering of vascular anatomy

Arteriography, a radiographic technique using invasive catheters to inject dye by puncturing the artery, does not satisfy the above criteria except for accurate anatomic and physiologic information. The advantage of sonography is that it is quick, painless and void of radiation. The physician can see tiny blood vessels in the body. Angiogenesis evaluation by power Doppler has proven clinically significant in providing important prognostic information in patients with colon, gastric, ovarian and cervical cancers and in malignant melanomas of the skin. Advantages (and disadvantages) are that it is both operator and equipment dependent. This requires a physician highly skilled in both ultrasound and urology for the prostate. The equipment varies widely in price and capability. Optimal equipment for the prostate has power Doppler and automated 3-D imaging features. Acceptable sonogram units can image blood vessels as small as 0.6 mm in diameter and show the capsule of the prostate in three dimensions. Units that can image blood vessels between 1.5 and 0.6 mm are important because the vascular nature of aggressive prostate cancer is that they are generally supplied by arteries within this size range.

Dr. William Lees of the University Medical College of London in 1994 described a paradox in prostate cancer imaging. The pathologist using a micro-scope showed cancers to be practically devoid of blood vessels or have very few feeding vessels. The sonogram in cancers depicts many blood vessels in high grade malignancies. The answer is that the pathologist sees micro-vessels in the cancer, and the sonogram sees the larger blood vessels required to feed the tumor.

Excellent quality images with CT angiography and MR angiography are available in many medical centers. No puncture of the artery is necessary, although the dye must be delivered by intravenous injection. Unfortunately, the vascular mapping of the prostate with this technique has not been fully studied. Other modalities such as contrast enhanced ultrasound, contrast enhanced CT, contrast enhanced MRI and diffusion MRI have not yet been clinically helpful in this area. My colleagues and I are testing a new MRI vascular computerized imaging protocol, called FTP MRI, which is proving useful. Thus far, it appears that the optimal way to diagnose aggressive prostate cancer is by using 3-D Power Doppler Sonography (3-D PDS). The major clinical use of combined 3-D PDS with FTP MRI is the assessment of therapy. We have found dramatic blood flow reductions in tumors within 2 weeks of treatment with these modalities. This visual confirmation as demonstrated by the book cover provides substantial psychological relief to the patient and often precludes the need for multiple biopsies.

Physicians in the United States may, in the near future, treat prostate cancer through the newer emerging technologies of endo (inside) vascular (vessel) therapy. European centers are injecting chemotherapies directly into the cancerous tissues rather than administering this toxic treatment throughout the body by intravenous injection. The results by Dr. Ursula Jacob in Germany have been impressive in many patients. Her cancer control has been verified by follow up with 3-D PDS and FTP MRI protocols as well as reduction of the PSA and clinical findings.

Dr. Barry Stein at the International Symposium on Endovascular Therapy, 2004 gave a lecture entitled, "New Concepts for a Modern Day Non-invasive Service" in which he claims that the report of a sonogram, CT or MR exam should contain a clinical assessment, including implications for possible endovascular management and treatment of the clinical problem. He feels that it is incumbent on the physician who images a cancer to offer the patient the benefit of the newer technologies over existing modalities.

He says:

We would be remiss if we didn't and couldn't educate the general public and patients to safer and less expensive alternative technologies to investigate disease…Patients are naturally very receptive to embrace any pain free, cutting edge technology over old relatively morbid alternatives. It is extremely important to empower the patient with the knowledge of alternative diagnostic studies when faced with the need for an angiogram (arterial dye study).

Said another way, the doctor who diagnoses the tumor could be the one to pursue treating it most effectively. It seems reasonable that the physician looking at a vascular prostate cancer would be the physician treating it. Logically, the tumor with high blood flow can be destroyed by cutting off the blood flow. The artery supplying the tumor can be identified and occluded in some mechanical fashion. It has been true that reduction or absence of tumor blood flows can be quickly assessed by 3-D PDS and/or FTP MRI.

So, how can one plug a blood vessel? Every housewife knows that there are two ways to block a sink drain. First, shove something big inside the pipe, which will block flow immediately. Another way is to flush small sticky food particles, like greasy rice and corn down the drain, which slowly obstructs it. Think of the hose supply a garden faucet as the artery that delivers blood to a cancer. A large object inside the artery will stop the flow at once. Smaller particles may not block the larger artery but will clog the smaller branches of the artery. In medicine, this process is called "embolization." This procedure has been successfully performed in Europe in prostate cancer treatments.

Another way to stop blood circulation to a tumor is to prevent the vessels from developing. This is like tying a tourniquet around the artery. Angiogenesis is a process where a tumor sends out protein molecules to promote development of new blood vessels. These vessels then provide nourishment to the cancer, even as they allow malignant cells to spread throughout the body. The recently FDA approved colon cancer drug **Avastin** cuts off the supply line to the tumor. This "antiangiogenesis" effect was discovered accidentally after the horrible birth defects from the pill, Thalidomide and was attributed to the observation that this drug blocked blood vessel growth in the developing fetus. There are over 70 antiangio-genesis drugs currently in human cancer testing. Although devastating to the unborn baby, these medications rarely cause significant side effects in older individuals. According to William Li, President of the Angiogenesis Foundation in Cambridge, the notorious drug, Thalidomide or its less toxic variants, may be the next product to receive FDA approval for stopping tumor growth.

My colleague, Dr. Federico Guercini, presented a paper at the 2005 AUA Meeting looking at the effect of Thalidomide in treating BPH. The initial results showed little improvement for the patient. However, a paper presented by Taiwanese radiologists, Dr. Chiun Hsu and associates, at the 2005 Radiologic Society of North America Meeting looked at the effect of Thalidomide on vascular liver tumors. Thalidomide has been intensively investigated as an anti-angiogenesis agent and proven effective in treating patients with multiple myeloma (common bone cancer in elderly patients) and Kaposi's sarcoma (aggressive skin malignancy common in AIDS patients). The author, Dr. Hsu, previously reported that low doses of Thalidomide induced a tumor control in patients with the highly vascular hepatocellular carcinoma (HCC or highly aggressive liver cancer). Dr. Hsu chose to follow treatments with Thalidomide by using power Doppler sonography (PDS) without the 3D component. In his series of 44 patients treated with oral thalidomide, 5 patients responded with clinically significant results. Of these responders, most had highly vascular tumors. The positive results of this study may be further enhanced in the liver and other organs by additional contemporaneous treatments such as RFA and HIFU or with other regional therapies. A downside to Thalidomide is the occurrence of deep venous thrombosis (blood clots in the veins that may go to the lungs) and peripheral neuropathy (nerve damage) that may be irreversible.

Studies are ongoing to decrease these side effects by adding other drugs in combination. The addition of heparin (blood thinner) has improved patient tolerance as reported in the *Journal of Clinical Oncology,* July 2004 issue. A study by the National Cancer Institute, by Dr. A. Retter and colleagues, suggested that this treatment would be optimally utilized in patients who have failed standard hormone treatments. Their paper presented at the 2005 Meeting of the American Society of Clinical Oncology, showed the entire patient group in the trial sustained PSA declines by greater than 50%. Thalidomide is currently marketed under the brand name THALOMID. Newer varieties of this drug with fewer side effects are currently being developed. Other novel therapies inhibiting blood vessel formation currently being studied are: Avastin, Celebrex, Cilengitide, Sorafenib and m-TOR inhibitors such as RAD001. It appears that combinations of drugs are more potent than single agents used alone.

Recent experience with other agents is shows blood vessel reduction of clinical value. Patients injected with botulinum neurotoxin by itself or in combination with other therapies are demonstrating significant decrease in tumor vascularity in both breast and prostate cancers. High doses of Co-enzyme Q 10 administered with antioxidants and plant sterols have reduced the blood vessel count in high grade cancers within a period of 2-3 weeks. This success, documented by radiologic imaging studies, gives the patient the assurance to continue on with this type of non invasive treatment. The new BPH drug, Avodart (dutasteride), has been anecdotally reducing blood flows in cancers as well as in benign enlargement. Dr. Ives, in 2005 *RADIOLOGY,* notes the blood flow reduction in benign disease is sufficient to highlight the tumor vessels in adjacent cancers. Further study of this pharmaceutical, according to Dr. Naslund, one of the early investigators, may show cancercidal effects. Of course, since this is in the same family as Proscar, which eventually proved to increase high grade tumors, more research must be obtained.

Microspheres are small beads that were first used in 1960 to block abnormal blood vessels in the brain. New microspheres of uniform size were developed in the mid 1990's to block dilated blood vessels and for preoperative embolization and devascularization of hypervascular tumors. The targeted embolization of benign uterine tumors (fibroids) has become an accepted treatment. Tagging chemotherapeutics or radioactive materials to these spheres has produced good clinical results in liver cancers of the primary type and metastatic variety. Japanese physicians have used this technique for the last 20 years. The studies on uterine tumors showed that the dilated feeding blood vessels preferentially suck up the microspheres in what is technically called the "sump effect." German physicians are using these effectively in prostate cancer control.

A variation on this concept is being developed in Montreal at the Laboratoire de Nanorobotique (Nanorobotic Laboratory) using magnetized microparticles (nano=extremely tiny particles). Magnetic nanospheres may be directed using MRI fields to position these "cluster time-bombs" inside the tumor. Radiofrequency waves of different types would activate them to produce local heat or release chemotherapeutics thereby destroying the cancer.

In 2004, the FDA approved Microcatheters, tiny tubes that are easier to use to deliver the payload to a tumor. They deliver medications, microspheres or a stent balloon to the renegade blood supply with minimal damage to the arterial system through which it passes. This is also a possible delivery system for drugs such as Thalidomide with its anti-angiogenesis capabilities. A special variation of this is called the stiletto catheter. This is designed to penetrate the wall of a blood vessel and inject chemical products or thermal destructive energies into a tumor bed. The medical name is locoregional therapy, since it uses the artery as a conduit to the tumor and then performs ablative therapy on the cancer tissue outside the artery. This work has been successfully performed on liver tumors at The Johns Hopkins Hospital. Locoregional ablative therapy uses one or a combination of percutaneous ethanol injections (alcohol), radiofrequency ablation (heat), microwave energy (heat), laser beams (heat), cryotherapy (cold), high intensity focused ultrasound (HIFU) and acids such as acetic acid.

MICROWAVE HYPERTHERMIA

Microwave hyperthermia is a non-ionizing form of radiation therapy that can substantially improve results from cancer treatment. In Phase III clinical trials where hypothermia was combined with ionizing radiation treatments, hyperthermia improved 2-year local control of melanoma from 28% to 46%, complete response for recurrent breast cancer from 38% to 60%, 2-year survival for glioblastoma (aggressive brain cancer) from 15% to 31% and complete response for advanced cervical cancer from 57% to 83%, as compared to the use of ionizing radiation therapy alone.

Vulnerability of cancerous tumors is a feature to be considered. Cancerous tumors are growths of mutated cells that often require far more energy to survive than do normal cells. As cancer cells multiply unchecked, they can quickly outstrip the capacity of their existing blood vessels to supply enough oxygen and nutrients to support them. In response, malignant tumors stimulate growth of additional blood vessels. However, these new blood vessels are mutated chaotic structures, as compared to blood vessels of normal tissues—of odd sizes, with loops and even blind ends. Because of this irregular blood vessel structure and rapid tumor growth, there are often large areas in tumors where the blood supply is deficient.

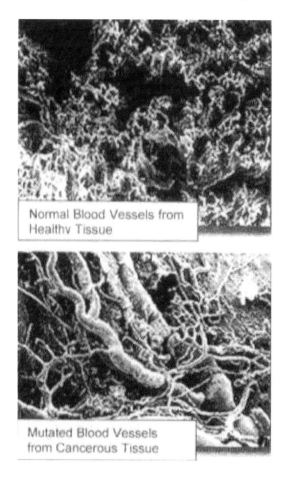

Normal Blood Vessels from Healthy Tissue

Mutated Blood Vessels from Cancerous Tissue

Cancerous tumors that do not have an adequate blood supply become oxygen starved (hypoxic) because blood is the source of oxygen delivery for cells. They also become acidic because hypoxic tumors cannot adequately expel waste through the blood. These tumors can even experience wide fluctuations in blood flow as their unstable blood vessels periodically collapse, making them acutely oxygen deficient for periods of time. Oxygen starved cancer cells are difficult to kill with ionizing radiation (which creates oxygen radicals that attack tumor DNA) or chemotherapy (where blood transport is required to deliver the drug). Destroying blood/oxygen depleted cancer is a very high priority in cancer therapy because hypoxic cancer cells are especially dangerous, prone to metastasize and spread the cancer to other parts of the body. The potentiating effect of botulinum neurotoxin in the cancercidal effects noted to occur with radiation and chemotherapy may be due to the opening of the arteries in the neighborhood of the tumor thereby increasing the oxygenation of the tissues.

Hyperthermia destroys cancer cells by raising the tumor temperature to a "high fever" range, similar to the way the body uses fever naturally when combating other forms of disease. Because the body's means of dissipating heat is through cooling from blood circulation, sluggish or irregular blood flow leaves cancerous tumors vulnerable to destruction at elevated temperatures that are safe for surrounding healthy tissues with normal, efficient blood cooling systems.

Scientists attribute the destruction of cancer cells at hyperthermic temperatures to damage in the cell membrane and the cell nucleus. Cancer cells are vulnerable to hyperthermia therapy particularly due to their high acidity caused by the inability to properly expel waste created by anaerobic (cellular) metabolism. Hyperthermia attacks acidic cells, disrupting the stability of cellular proteins and killing them. Hyperthermia is proving effective in increasing the effectiveness of radiation therapy, chemotherapy and surgery, since tumors tend to shrink after this treatment.

Gene therapy research is showing hyperthermia to be an activator to turn on new biological therapies, speeding gene production by thousands of times (heat mediated gene therapy). Hyperthermia plays an essential role in the development of anti-tumor vaccines that are based on heat shock patients. Research is showing hyperthermia to be an angiogenesis inhibitor, preventing cancer from inducing growth of new blood vessels to expand its blood supply.

Hyperthermia has further demonstrated use as a companion therapy for drug angiogenesis inhibitors, used in the final destruction of depleted cancer cells that survive blood starved conditions. Gene therapy for treating the deadly vascular tumor, malignant melanoma, was successful in 2 out of 17 patients, in a study by the National Cancer Institute. Leukocytes (white blood cells) were infused with cancer killing virus genes and injected intravenously. Perhaps the addition of hyperthermia, botulinum neurotoxin injection and intra-arterial targeted delivery would increase the effectiveness of this type of therapy.

Hyperthermia has improved Quality of Life parameters for many patients. A recent study by the National Academy of Sciences has pointed out the shortcomings of the single-minded search for cancer cure while ignoring existing patients who need treatment for pain and other conditions associated with cancer. A substantial improvement in both palliation and durability of palliation has been observed when hyperthermia is added to ionizing radiation treatments. Some scientists have noted that hyperthermia stimulates the immune system, assisting patients in recovery from toxic cancer therapies such as chemotherapy and ionizing radiation. Even in situations where there is no hope for survival, hyperthermia may provide benefit through alleviation of such effects as bleeding, pain and infection.

Over the past fifteen years there have been 33 published clinical trials (17 Phase I or II and 16 Phase III) on the effects of hyperthermia combined with ionizing radiation, chemotherapy or both. The following published studies completed at notable research centers in North America and Europe are amongst the most significant:

In 1993 the *International Journal of Radiation Oncology, Biology, Physics* reported the results of a 41 patient (44 node) Phase III clinical trial involving inoperable Stage IV head and neck cancer conducted by Drs. Valdagni and Amichelli at the Institute of Science and Technology at Ricerca, Italy. The study concluded that hyperthermia added to ionizing radiation improved complete response from 41% to 83%, local relapse-free survival from 24% to 68% and overall survival at 5 years from 0% to 53%, as compared to ionizing radiation treatments alone.

In 1996 the *International Journal of Hyperthermia* reported the results of Phase III clinical trials on 128 tumors involving recurrent or metastatic malignant melanoma as conducted by Dr. Overgaard and colleagues performed at the Danish Cancer Society University Hospital in Denmark. The study concluded that the addition of hyperthermia to ionizing radiation increased the complete response rate of recurrent malignant melanoma lesions from 35% to 62%, and local relapse-free survival at five years from 28% to 46%, as compared to ionizing radiation treatments alone.

In 1996 the *International Journal of Radiation Oncology, Biology, Physics* reported the results of a 306 patient Phase III clinical trial involving superficial localized breast cancer conducted by Vernon and colleagues at Hammersmith Hospital. The study concluded that the addition of hypothermia to ionizing radiation increased complete response from 41% to 59% and local relapse-free survival from 30% to 50%.

In 1996 the International Journal of the American Cancer Society, *Cancer,* reported the results of a 23 patient clinical trail involving carcinoma of the head and neck region, carcinoma of the breast and malignant melanoma, conducted by Drs. Lee, Mayer and Hallinan of Johns Hopkins Hospital. The study produced complete response in 89% of patients and partial response in 11% of patients, with a two-year actuarial local control rate of 74% using interstitial hypothermia in combination with radioactive seeds (brachytherapy). The study concluded that "outpatient interstitial thermoradiotherapy is convenient, safe, and efficacious for treating human neoplasms."

In 1998 the *International Journal of Radiation Oncology, Biology, Physics* reported the results of a 112 patient Phase III clinical trial involving glioblastoma multi-forme (aggressive brain cancer) conducted by Sneed and colleagues at the University of California, San Francisco. The study showed a more than double two-year survival rate using brachytherapy plus hyperthermia as compared to brachytherapy alone.

In 1999 the *International Journal of Radiation Oncology, Biology, Physics* reported the results of a 97 patient Phase III clinical trial involving high-grade soft tissue sarcomas conducted by Dr. Prosnitz at Duke University Medical Center in North Carolina. This study showed excellent local control of extremity lesions (95% control) when hyperthermia was combined with radiation. (German clinical trials have also reported that hyperthermia enhances the effectiveness of certain chemotherapy drugs, even in drug-resistant cells, when treating locally advanced sarcomas (malignant soft tissue tumors).

In 2000 *The Lancet* reported results of a 358 patient Phase III clinical trial involving locally advanced pelvic tumors that was conducted by Dr. van der Zee and the Dutch Hyperthermia Group at University Hospital Cancer Center in Rotterdam. The study reported that hyperthermia in combination with ionizing radiation improved complete response rates for bladder cancer 51% to 73%, complete response rates for advanced cervical cancer from 57% to 83%, and overall three-year survival from 27% to 51%.

Chemoembolization is a commonly performed procedure in liver cancers which uses two concepts of blood flow physiology. First, blood brings chemother-apeutic agents into the cancer bed. Secondly, blocking or embolization of the blood supply reduces delivery of oxygen to the tumor and prevents a normal blood flow to wash away the chemotherapeutic drugs. Average hospital stay is 36 hours and complications are low. The median survival rate of 26 months is the same result as surgically treated tumors.

Combining two minimally invasive interventional radiology treatments for liver cancer is as effective as surgery for treating single tumors up to seven centimeters in diameter, according to new data presented at the 2004 annual meeting of the Society of Interventional Radiology and the 2006 World Congress of Interventional Oncology. Many studies of combination therapies have begun in 2005 and initial results are encouraging for prostate cancers.

The treatment combines embolization (blocking the blood supply to the tumor), with radiofrequency ablation (killing the tumor with heat). This combination is effective at treating solitary hepatocellular carcinoma (virulent liver tumor) lesions up to seven centimeters and affords patients survival benefits on par with surgical resection but without the trauma, according to the study. The minimally invasive interventional treatment targets only the tumor tissue and spares the healthy tissue. It also offers an easier and much quicker recovery than surgery. At the 2006 meeting of physicians and engineers from the IEEE in New York by The Glaucoma Foundation, the possibility of iron particles coated with chemotherapies could be guided by MRI or other magnetic fields anywhere in the body in a targeted manner to kill tumors. Once in position, these armored warriors could be induced to release their toxic packages locally, thus sparing the body the major side effects of chemotherapy.

"This new treatment takes two well-established interventional radiology procedures and combines them to optimize treatment for patients with primary liver cancer, "says study investigator Anne Covey, M.D., an interventional radiologist at Memorial Sloan Kettering Cancer Center in New York. She iterates, "Although surgical resection has historically been considered the gold standard for the treatment of patients with single lesions, the survival data for the combined treatments is promising, and we remain cautiously optimistic that these results will hold up in the long term."

The January 2005 issue of *Radiology Today* quotes Dr. Charles Cantor on genetic treatment of breast and prostate cancer, both of which are hormonally dependent and look similar under the microscope. Dr. Cantor cites the December 2004 issue of *Cancer Research* that shows individuals with a certain bad gene have a 40 percent higher chance of developing breast and prostate cancer compared to those without this genetic defect. While the original study was designed to track breast cancer, it was found that it held true for prostate tumors. Since the bad genes are on the cell surface, Dr Cantor predicts that new therapeutic opportunities will arise for breast and prostate cancer patients as drugs are made to target these sites.

NEW MRI BLOOD FLOW TECHNOLOGIES

Given the high specificity of cancer detection by abnormal blood flows by 3D PDS, the MRI researchers have been improving blood flow techniques that point out tumors. My colleagues and I have been studying various blood flow enhancers over the past 24 months. The early indicators of tumor growth were disappointing and much effort has gone into developing a better class of computer software analysis. The essence of MRI detection of cancer is "leaky vessels", that is, abnormal vessels leak the injectable media which marks the tumor tissues. The latest protocols have been highly successful in demonstrating the cancer and its extracapsular spread and were reported in the 2007 conference of the *American Roentgen Ray Society* by Drs. Bard, Liebeskind and Melnick and by myself at the 2007 *American Society of Clinical Oncology.* A few cases of boney tumor metastases have detected with a specificity exceeding standard MRI results and will be followed and reported in the next edition of this book.

Recent articles combining the use of *quercitin, resveratrol* and *ellagic acid* with localized hyperthermia are proving helpful in treatment of boney metastases. Hyperthermic states may be achieved simply by the use of therapeutic ultrasound units that treat muscle and pain disorders or more accurately by advanced radio or microwave generators. Dr. Paliwal, in the 2005 *British Journal of Cancer,* notes pretreatment of prostate cancer with ultrasound hyperthermia dramatically increases cell cancer death caused by the simultaneous administration of *quercitin.*

IRREVERSIBLE ELECTROPORATION (IRE)

Dr. Gary Onik, at the 2006 Annual Symposium of Interventional Therapy and the 2006 World Congress of Interventional Oncology, unveiled a novel ablation technique that uses non thermal electromagnetic waves and may be competitive with current thermal ablation methodologies. This modality is undergoing approval by the FDA and will be available for selected patients in 2007. The process is rapid and appears not to affect adjacent non cancerous structures such as nerves, bowel and bladder. The patented technology ablates a zone that can be imaged by 3D PDS as an echo poor zone (dark) that turns echogenic (white) in 24 hours. This finding has not been confirmed by CT and MRI modalities. A suprising finding was that treated tumors produced an enhanced immunologic response to combat disease at the metastatic sites of the tumor.

DENDRITIC CELL IMMUNOTHERAPY

Immunotherapy uses the natural cellular immune system of the body to defend itself. The immune system consists of anatomic barriers such as the skin and acid in the stomach. If a foreign substance penetrates this shield, a second line defense is the inflammatory response. The last line of defense is the immune system which uses white blood cells to attack the invading organism.

White blood cells include neutrophils which kill bacteria, eosinophils involving delayed response, monocytes (also called macrophages) which are scavengers and lymphocytes which transfer cellular information and produce antibodies which inactivate or destroy foreign cells. When a tumor cell is noticed by the immune system, first a monocyte attaches and begins to digest the cell by breaking it into little pieces. The monocyte will then hand off the tumor remnants to other cells or transform itself into a specialized immune cell called a dendritic cell. This cell then migrates to a nearby lymph node which activate the army of lymphocytes (cytotoxic T lymphocytes) that attack the surface membrane of the cancer cells.

To be effective, the dendritic cell must be mature. Researchers are successfully completing this task and there have been studies showing its effectiveness in combating prostate cancer, lymphoma and malignant melanoma. At a 2006 think tank on evolving cancer therapies in New York, a highly successful treatment on prostate cancer patients was reported performed in the Phillipines. The treatment seems to have few side effects and will be carefully monitored by the medical community. It is not FDA approved and is currently being performed outside the United States in several centers with good results.

NANOPARTICLE THERMAL ABLATION

Another spin-off of a military technology is now being applied to patient treatment. A battlefield repair system for body armor and other composite materials uses a resin saturated with nanoparticles (as many as 10,000 can fit on the end of a pin) that become heated when exposed to a magnetic field. The heated resin was molded and used to patch the broken materials before it cooled. The 2007 *Journal of Nuclear Medicine* cited an article by Dr. Gerald DeNardo and a world wide group of authors participating in a UC Davis Medical School study of treatment of tumors in animals using this technique of heating in combination with nanoparticles labeled with antibodies specific to breast cancer cells. In the lab studies, it was found breast cancer cells were specifically killed when the culture dishes were exposed to antibody labeled iron oxide particles and an alternating magnetic field. For the non physicist readers, think of the new teapots that use electricity to generate heat inside the container while the outside remains cool. They were designed for blind people' safety when handling boiling water. After injection trillions of nanoparticles of antibody-iron oxide and waiting three days for accumulation in the targeted cancer, magnetic fields instantly generated heat sufficient to kill the tumor without damaging nearby structures. Particles outside the tumor field were not significantly heated during the 20 minutes of treatment. No treatment side effects or toxicity was noted. It was felt that the treatment could be used to safely treat tumors anywhere in the body, as long as the circulating antibody-nanoparticle entity could get there. Since there is blood flow to all tumors, it would not matter where the cancer is located. Human engineered antibodies exist for breast, prostate, lung, colon and ovarian cancers. Also, lymph node metastases from malignant melanoma and breast cancer could be targeted.

NANOPARTICLE CHEMOTHERAPY

An interesting property of microbubbles (water coated tiny air pockets) is that they may be made to rupture under a burst of ultrasound energy. This means that microbubbles may be steered into a tumor and then exploded by targeted sonography. Researchers at the University Hospital of Utah have been coating these objects with nanoparticles containing chemotherapeutic agents and permeating cancers with focal treatments. This work is encouraging and other similar pinpoint nanoparticle therapies are currently being developed with MRI technologies.

CHEMOSENSITIVITY TESTING AND CHEMOEMBOLIZATION

Low dose targeted chemotherapy is possible if the right drug can be put in the right place. Dr. Ursula Jacob, of the Leonardis Klinic in Germany, has been using a blood assay to show the metabolic pathway of the cancer on a molecular-genetic basis. If a particular pathway is active, then it is more likely a chemotherapeutic agent based on this pathway will be effective. The test analyses and identifies circulating tumor cells in the blood stream. The test is only effective if circulating tumor cells are present. Also studied are the activity of the natural killer (NK) cells and modalities to increase their effectiveness. Based on these results, localized or whole body hyperthermia may be induced at the time the chemoembolic agents are injected into the artery feeding the tumor. High concentrations may be focally delivered sparing the normal tissues producing greater clinical outcome and fewer side effects.

GENE THERAPY / MOLECULAR BIOLOGY

In previous chapters, the future of genetic "bullets" looked promising, however, a four year study from the United States Human Genome Research Institute (involving 80 organizations around the world) is reshaping our mile posts. The long held view was each single gene in living organisms (humans, animals, plants, bacteria) carried the information essential to construct a single protein specific to that molecule. Proteins are the building blocks and power systems that regulate cells, and by extension, living organisms. In the 60's, scientists discovered that a gene that produced one type of protein in one organism would produce a very close molecular clone in another entity. The standard medical application of this feature enabled insulin from pigs to be used safely by humans in the treatment of diabetes. It was assumed for years that a gene from a donor of any organism would predictably produce specified functions in another host organism. It was hoped genetic therapies would have a uniform effect with clear boundaries and discrete properties. Researchers depended on the fact that each sequence of DNA was linked to a single medical application, such as a predisposition to cancer, heart disease or diabetes.

The conclusion of this study by 35 international research groups showed a complex network of interactions between gene that is casting doubt on the "one gene, one protein" postulation. The assumption that genes operated independently must be rethought since overlapping functions of genetic material were shown to occur as the norm rather than as the exception. Genes are only one component of how a genome functions, with the other components not clearly understood. It seems that diseases are caused not by the action of a single gene, but rather by the interaction of multiple genes. Specifically, a virulent form of malaria appears to involve interactions of 500 genes. It is hoped that another conclave of scientists will provide a clinical application manual for the newly discovered genetic variants in human treatment.

PHOTODYNAMIC THERAPY OR CYTOLUMINECENT THERAPY

The use of light in the treatment of cancer, developed in the late 19th century in Germany, underwent a revival when the Japanese treated lung cancers in the 1980's. In 1998, the FDA approved this modality for microinvasive lung tumors. The patient is first given an intravenous injection of a photosensitizer, which selectively accumulates in cancerous tissues. A laser beam is directed at the lung tumor produces a free radical oxygen molecule that internally destroys tumor cells. This is considered a less invasive procedure than surgery and can be repeated without systemic toxicity.

Reports of successful light treatments of sensitized prostate cancer tissue have appeared sporadically. Dr. Nathan, in 2002 *Journal of Urology*, effectively treated local recurrence in a small study of radiotherapy failures, however, 4 of the 14 patients developed incontinence. Another side effect is the uptake by the photosensitizer in all the tissues rendering patients acutely light sensitive for up to 6 weeks. Additionally, the light has to be directly applied to the tumor by fiberoptic cables, necessitating sedation or general anesthesia.

I have seen some post treatment failures in my practice and some apparent initial successes as demonstrated by the change in tumor vascularity by 3D PDS. A study by Drs. Pendse and Allen of the University College London presented at the 2007 AUA meeting looked at a novel photosensitizer and follow up post-treatment using CE-MRI. Tookad is a new light activated drug developed at Israel's Weitzman Institute of Science. 27 patients were primed with injected Tookad (WST-09) after MRI delineated their biopsy proven tumors. Light was diffused into the prostate under general anesthesia. CE-MRI taken one week post-therapy showed absent flow in the treatment sites which were followed up to 6 months. Long term studies will show the overall effectiveness of this modality.

GALVANOTHERAPY (GT) AND ELECTROCHEMOTHERAPY (ECT)
Named in honor of the Italian pioneer in electricity, Luigi Galvani, this low voltage DC current therapy is a form of minimally invasive treatment used primarily in Germany and Scandinavia. The voltage used is similar to a 9 volt battery and in the skin produces connective tissue formation and destroys malignancies by a combination of physical change and acceleration of immunologic activity at the tumor site.

FUTURE RESEARCH
The nature of honest medical investigation is that suprises often occur. Innovation is risky. The art of medical innovation is to generate new uses for the unexpected. Simply put, "When life hands you a lemon, take sugar and ice and make lemonade" It is hoped that researchers will have the integrity to identify early side effects as well as lateral possibilities of their discoveries. Proponents of a discovery and have tunnel vision regarding the benefits of their product. Many drugs approved by the FDA and hyped on television commercials have been pulled off the market as life threatening problems became too apparent to dismiss.

Some dangerous outcomes have taken half a century in their development. For example, the drug Penicillin that saved my life as a child with pneumonia eventually led to the creation of "superbugs" that are virtually unkillable. How did this happen? Antibiotics were truly miracle drugs that destroyed microbes. Not well understood for years was the genetic material responsible for conferring antibiotic resistance passed easily between different types of bacteria. The overprescribing of antibiotics for every ailment, especially the common "cold" which is viral in nature, has created germs that are resistant to a class of antibiotic treatments. This development led to development of ever more powerful types of antibiotics which resulted in more varieties of stronger bacteria. We are at a point where some bacteria are more powerful than the existing pharmaceutical products. While no one could envision this scenario, hindsight offers researchers the perspective of vigilance in monitoring the effects of their creations.

Unexpected positive side effects may occur when men taking antioxidant preparations notice healthier skin in addition to improved tumor response. Another surprising consequence was their medicine began disappearing too quickly. It turned out that their wives started using the herbal formulations to attain smoother skin for themselves. Unexpected negative side effects occurred with the early use of MRI. In the breast the number of false positives was greater than 50% for years and in the prostate it approximated 30%. Newer contrast protocols have improved this greatly.

Patients, the end users of modern technology, can be helpful in documenting and reporting unusual happenings. The team of patient, physician and scientist together can build a healthier future for mankind. Proven technologies may be further developed while problematic modalities may be ear-marked for overhaul or discard before they produce more harm to the public. Also, many medical discoveries are published daily in prestigious scientific journals or presented at major specialty conferences without these findings made available to the general public. The sheer volume of new findings has inundated physicians and confused patients. Our challenge is to ferret out important ideas and bring these to the attention of the medical community and patients likely to benefit from the treatment. Medical history demonstrates that administrative committees do not make discoveries-breakthroughs occur when individuals committed to change think outside the box and work outside the prevailing dogmatic principles. To paraphrase a quote: We will not have the land of the free if we are not the home of the brave. Re-stated, that means we must take risks and innovate if we are to fully harvest the fruits of scientific research.

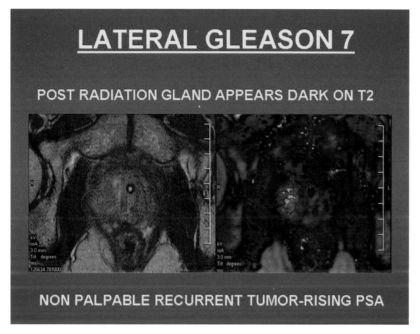

Fig. 9.2 Colorization of abnormality on standard MRI improves diagnostic accuracy

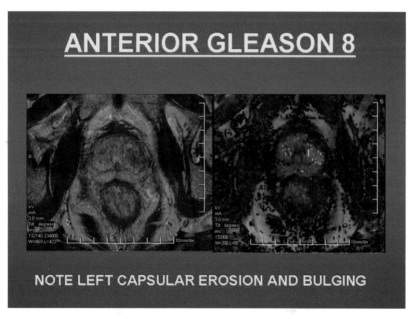

Fig. 9.3 Color coding improves diagnosis of tumor spread through capsule

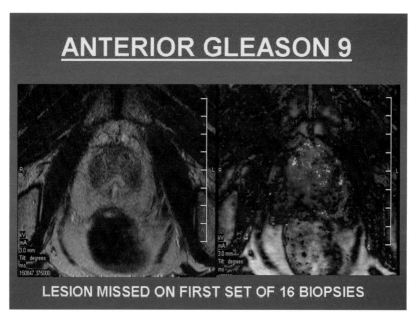

Fig. 9.4 Anterior tumor confirmed when biopsy performed under ultrasound guidance

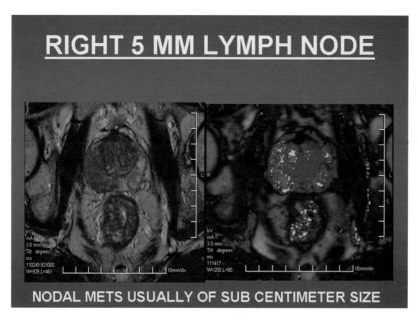

Fig 9.5 Lymph node metastases usually less than 1 cm and may be missed by CT scans

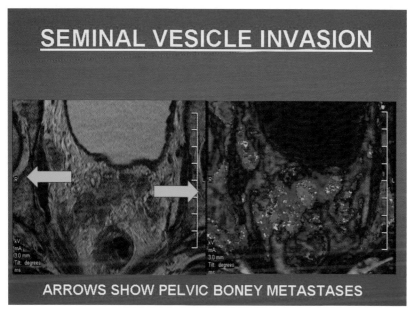

Fig 9.6 Tumor extension to seminal vesicles above prostate gland is well imaged by MRI

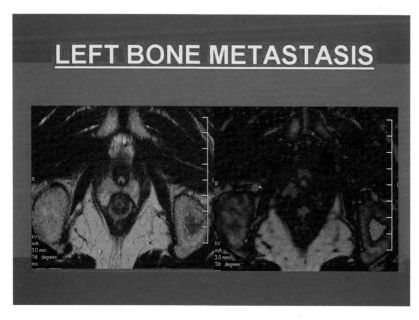

Fig 9.7 Single bone metastasis clearly detected on colorized MRI (left)

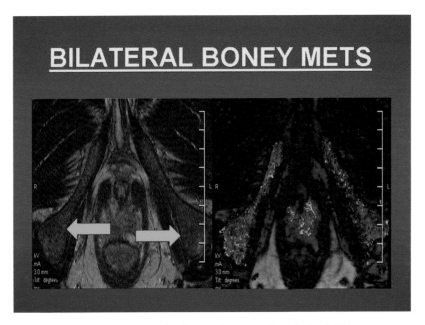

Fig 9.8 Bone metastases (red) are diagnosed early by MRI imaging

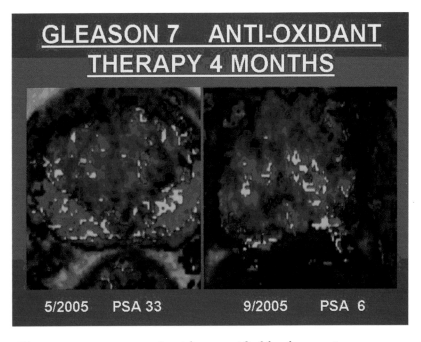

Fig 9.9 Treatment success on anti-oxidants verified by decrease in tumor vascularity

CHAPTER TEN
Cancer Screening Pro's and Con's

Screening is hot business-hot, for patients, because they get their fears resolved, and, business for providers, since their business is booming. Early detection of serious disease, such as coronary artery disease with electron beam computed tomography (EBCT-special CT scan showing calcification of the arteries to the heart) and screening for lung cancer with computed tomography (CT-scans) is commonplace and rising in popularity even though there is no proven reduction in mortality from these diseases by earlier discovery. Not only are these studies controversial, it is unclear at this time whether the potential benefits outweigh the risks. Risks, such as unnecessary workups for false positive test results, excessive cost of "downstream" procedures, false reassurance from false negative results, are common. Risks from radiation and patient anxiety have not been fully assessed at this time. Yet, patients are paying out of pocket and physicians are referring for these exams. People pay for "peace of mind"

What can be done in the present environment of high demand and lax physician oversight? Education of both patients and physicians may be initiated in the format of informed decision making (IDM) and shared decision making (SDM). Is it appropriate to offer an unproven screening test before it has been proved through clinical trials? Is it wise to deny a patient access to a screening that may give them relief from anxiety? Stress and anxiety are proven killers. Many cancers are not lethal. The vast majority of men would rather be told they have a prostate cancer-thus providing a resolution to their fear's-rather than not being sure and living in uncertainty. Almost all women breathe an audible sigh of relief when I tell them their mammogram is negative and their breast sonogram is benign. Probably the worst effect of a false positive screening test is the undue worry about the effect of the disease on oneself and one's family. A secondary bad effect is the hassle and costs in terms of time and money of the unending follow up downstream tests to confirm the screening possibility.

What about the early detection of a disease for which there need be no treatment? In this case, ignorance is not only bliss, it is useful. What about the early detection of a problem from which there is no treatment? Perhaps ignorance cannot hurt in the long run. Early detection may not mean better care, either. In the case of removal of a small tumor detected by screening that leaves behind the parent and larger malignancy that may have been found by standard medical care at a later interval, the patient has been disserved by earlier diagnosis. There is also a financial drain on the health care system when a screening turns up the need for additional testing and treatments. The deliverer of the screening may wish to educate the patient as to the unproven nature of the test and the potential risks associated with the procedure. For example, when patients learn the 97% accuracy of serious prostate cancer discovered by the combination of 3D-PDS and MRI, many defer the biopsy which offers less than a 50–50 chance of confirmation in most patients. The possibility of a biopsy spreading the tumor is also foremost on the minds of most patients, even though their surgeons have down played this possibility. Many patients also rethink their treatment options when learning of the high rates of cancer recurrence following standard tumor therapy regimens. In fact, a study by Braddock in a 1999 issue of the *Journal of the American Medical Association* showed only 9% of patients met the criteria for IDM in the 3552 clinical decisions reviewed.

The 2007 *Journal of the American College of Radiology* defines 10 criteria for screening tests:

1. The disease has serious consequences.
2. The screening population has a high prevalence of detectable preclinical phase
3. The test detects little pseudodisease: disease that would not become clinically significant: a)non progressive disease b)progressive, but not clinically significant
4. High accuracy in finding the detectable preclinical phase
5. Detecting disease before the critical point of clinical injury
6. Low morbidity
7. Test is affordable and available
8. Treatment exists
9. Treatment is more effective when applied before symptoms begin
10. Treatment is not too risky or toxic

The American College of Physicians has set forth a charter on the ethics of unproven screening tests that requires the physician to empower his or her patient to make informed decisions. IDM, informed decision making, includes the possible side effects of the tests, the accuracy and limitations inherent in the exam and the alternatives to the procedure including doing nothing. Screening options are also more complex with the rapid technological advances in the first five years of the 21st century. For colorectal cancer screening, patients may choose from the following menu: colonoscopy (entire colon), flexible sigmoidoscopy (lower colon), air-contrast barium enema (x ray study using air in an enema), fecal occult blood testing (detects blood in stool from bleeding tumor) and virtual colonoscopy (CT scans of inside of colon). Patients must consider the risks and benefits of the PSA test for prostate cancer. Controversies still exist over the age to start mammograms and how often women should get Pap smears for cervical cancer. Patients, now more than ever, want to participate in their own care. Patients want a relationship with their physician based on mutual participation.

The widespread dissemination of accurate health information on the Internet and through dedicated cancer support groups gives patients the right to share their knowledge and informed opinions with those of their physician's. Indeed, much of what I have learned about alternative medicine comes from listening to the success stories of my patients. When I hear of some strange medicament helping someone I put it in the back of my mind. If I hear ten men tell similar experiences, I shift this concept to the front of my mind and raise my antennae to listen for more details. When I hear a hundred men recount similar experiences from an herb I had no knowledge of, I find out more from the Internet and research the medical databases. Case in point: I practiced Tai Chi for two years. This martial art focuses on balance, sensitivity and alertness. By using vision exercises developed in antiquity I was able to dramatically improve my peripheral vision. I actually avoided an automobile accident without being aware of it on a conscious level. One day I was driving towards the Queensboro Bridge in mid Manhattan when suddenly I swerved the steering wheel to the left and felt my heart flutter. I did not see the car about to hit me on the right. My newly acute peripheral visual input bypassed my mind and told my nervous system to get out of harm's way. When I told this to my ophthalmologist, he discounted my experience and solemnly warned me never to press on my eyeballs (something he knew affected patients who performed karate) since it could slow my heart and cause me to faint.

IDM occurs when the individual fully understands the nature and scope of the clinical service. That is, the expected outcome: likely consequences, including risks, limitations, benefits, alternatives and uncertainties. The patient must consider his preference as appropriate and feel he has fully participated in the decision making at a personally desirable level. IDM and SDM differ somewhat from legal informed consent. The legal medical consent is based upon the competence of both parties, full disclosure by the physician, understanding, voluntary agreement and lastly, consent by the patient. In contrast, IDM and SDM take into account the degree to which a patient may or may not choose to participate in a decision making process and focus on producing decisions consistent with patient' preferences and values.

Decision making is most important when there are several equal and valid tests available for the same medical problem. The patient must recognize that a test often involves more than a single encounter and the results frequently translate to a new medical journey upon which he must unwillingly travel. An article for radiologists in the *Journal of the American College of Radiology* in April 2005 asks diagnostic imagers who perform radiologic screening tests to learn from the lesson of the unproven PSA blood test. Citing evidence that there is no clear evidence that PSA screening reduces the mortality of prostate cancer, the American College of Physicians and the American Urological Association recommend that patients be informed of the know risks and potential benefits of PSA testing so they can make personal decisions about testing. The risks include further testing such as biopsy of the prostate from false positive results, unnecessary worry, and the side effects of common treatments (impotence and incontinence) when the natural course of the disease may not have affected a man's mortality.

One problem of testing is that up to one third of men who had PSA tests did not realize that was included in their testing series. This raises concern for the potential harm that may arise when men must cope with the consequences of a test they did not even know they had taken. The results of a simple test may lead to a cascade of future decisions about follow up testing and possibly various unpleasant treatments. While some argue the reassurance of a negative test results in a grateful patient, others note that the most aggressive prostate cancers do not make PSA and thus are not ruled out by a low or normal PSA level. Indeed, a European study of 2074 screening biopsies presented at the 100th American Urological Association Meeting by Drs. W. Horninger and G. Bartsch confirmed that the percentage of high grade (Gleason greater than or equal to 7) cancers was substantial. In the PSA group of 1–2, there were 13% of high grade tumors; in the PSA group of 2–3, there were 22% of high grade cancers, and, in the PSA group of 3–4, there were 22% of high grade cancers.

Dr. Klotz's article on active surveillance in chapter 7 also invites discussion of current screening concepts for prostate cancer. He notes "If all American men between 50–70 with PSA>2.5 had a biopsy…775,000 cases of cancer would be found…which is 25 times (2500% higher) than the 30,350 men expected to die of PC per year in the US." He quotes the 2004 *Canadian Cancer Journal* article by Jemal demonstrating the lifetime risk of dying from prostate cancer remaining less than 3%. His own phase III study is showing that aggressive treatment of PC improves survival for 1every out of 100 patients. He does not take in consideration the problem of interval cancers. As I stated in the 2006 *JFR* meeting, interval tumors are highly aggressive and occur within 6 months. This is why our group performs screening sonography of the breast and prostate at half yearly intervals. Our two year study showed about 5% of men developed high grade prostate tumors every 6 months which was clearly demonstrable by 3D PDS and confirmed by FTP MRI.

I implemented an IDM and SDM system in my office at the beginning of 2004. My patients are seated in front a computer and view a presentation of my tests and possible treatments with limitations and side effects so they can make their independent decision. During my testing, I show my patient exactly what I am seeing on a large overhead screen and especially highlight areas of concern and explain their nature. After my testing results are explained to my patient, I sit with him (and wife, if available) and we make shared decisions. I give my patients a preliminary report to read. I then go over what they understood with their family, if present, and what they choose to do for treatment. I also hand them a copy of their final report, a set of ultrasound images on a compact disc and a written sheet of paper listing all the possible treatments, with their side effects, including phone numbers of other specialists to whom they may speak directly.

Through the Biofoundation for Angiogenesis R&D, I have developed relationships with the world wide leaders in many areas of prostate medicine. Most have agreed to work together as a team to advance the state of prostate cancer treatment and personally advise patients courageous enough to consider alternative and probable future FDA approved treatments. These dedicated and busy physicians will, to make further breakthroughs in medicine, give of their time to confer with and support men trying to make a better life by taking a chance on promising new technologies. To paraphrase Mother Teresa, do a little good with a lot of love and eventually the world will be a better place. Tony Cointreau, who worked with Mother Teresa in India and became her trusted biographer, was presented as the 2005 Humanitarian Award winner in New York City. Upon the celebrity packed stage, he said: "The simple truth, starting with a whisper, kindled by hope, reinforced by courage, emboldened by commitment and strengthened by knowledge will evolve, triumph and impact the world like a comet."

I ask my patients, if they so wish, to consult their hearts, their minds, their family, their friends, their physicians and spiritual advisors and call me in a week or so to refine their decisions with me. Results by Dr. A. Wolf in the 1996 *Archives of Internal Medicine* noted that decision aids improved knowledge, decreased interest in PSA screening and increased interest and participation in the decision making process. An ethical approach to unproven screening tests being developed suggest health care providers fulfill the five components of informed consent with their patients:

1. assess a patient's competence to make a decision
2. disclose the key facts
3. make sure the patient understands by asking the patient what he heard
4. make sure the patient can make a voluntary decision
5. make sure the patient is able to give consent

An open ended question such as, "Tell me in your own words how you arrived at your decision, the risks and benefits you see, and the options you are considering" is a sentence I find helpful with my patients to establish and review their decision process. One problem in discussing options is the divide between the complex nature of medicine and the personal nature of and individual patient needs. In addition to asking men what their personal considerations are, I inform them of facts that previous patients have told me about quality of life issues that were not apparent until after the tests and treatments were undertaken, such as: after HIFU occasionally I would find fragments of my prostate in the urine, after hormones my hip fractured, after antioxidants I lost 15 pounds, on plant hormones my skin got better and my wife (and my mistress) started stealing my pills, etc. I then tailor my responses to individual concerns. For example, complaints I have heard about the post HIFU cancer treatment experience have included the need for a catheter to be worn in the penis for a few weeks. While most men accepted this as a necessary evil, one of my patients challenged me, saying he would risk the procedure without a catheter or he would not be treated at all. I discussed this option with my team and we came up with the alternative of placing a catheter in the bladder instead of inside the penis. This suprapubic (bladder) catheter worked so well on this patient, that it has now become the standard of post treatment HIFU care and actually improved the postoperative course by reducing the time for urination to return to normal on all patients and contributing greatly to patient comfort at the same time. According to the ethics guidelines of the American College of Radiology, since many patients are referred to me directly by friends and family, and not by other physicians, I am obligated to inform them of the risks, benefits and limitations of my testing. I request my patients and potential referring physicians look at my Web site www.cancerscan.com before and after they see me to be maximally informed and make any suggestions that may improve the informational content. I mention that my equipment is specifically calibrated to detect the 3% of cancer that is lethal and may not always detect some of the remaining 97% that is not overtly lethal and can be managed conservatively. I highlight studies from international medical centers showing that the 3D PDS is 95% accurate in detecting Gleason 7 or higher, may show seminal vesicle invasion and usually discerns extracapsular spread on the 3 Dimensional reconstruction and analysis of the 800 to 1400 images that are captured as a reference data set in the computer and studied on a radiologic 4-D workstation. When indicated by high suspicion of spread outside the capsule, I obtain an MRI which shows adjacent lymph nodes (glands) and metastases to bones and the adjacent seminal vesicles. The MRI is much more sensitive in this regard than the CT scan and has no radiation. The new computer aided MRI showing abnormal blood vessels combined with the 3D PDS has added greatly to the follow up of treated tumors. If suspicious lymph nodes are detected, the new *Combidex* MRI performed in Europe shows if the tumor has spread to the glands and which nodes are involved. My written material notes the combination of FTP-MRI and 3D-PDS is 97 % accurate in detecting significant cancers. Of greatest importance is the ability to demonstrate the response of a vascular tumor to therapy within a short period of time that provides patients with a milestone marker with which to better guide their treatment plan.

APPENDIX

Testimonials

August 4, 2005

Dear Dr. Bard:

On June 29, 2005 I went to see you. Thanks to your expertise and very special equipment which provides 3-D imaging, you found that I had a virulent type of prostate cancer. You gave me a packet of materials on HIFU treatment—high intensity focused ultrasound. The treatment's 90 degree Celsius temperature destroys the cancer cells in seconds without side effects. Clearly, this is a major breakthrough in prostate cancer treatment.

Shortly thereafter I saw my urologist who scoffed at your findings of virulence. He said emphatically that this could not be determined. Also that 97 percent of prostate cancers are benign. Especially, since I am 94, he advised me to sit tight. If the situation worsened badly, radiation could be used.

Radiation did not seem to me much of an option. It involves a considerable blood loss, and I have anemia and heart problems.

My Urologist's advice plainly was based on probability—that 97 percent of prostate cancers are benign. But probability doesn't apply to a single event, such as one case. His advice involved a gamble, one contrary to your findings that I was among the 3 percent: Speed in treatment was essential. HIFU is available only before the cancer has metastasized.

Time was not on my side. On July 31 I underwent treatment in Cancun, Mexico at an American Hospital. My doctor George M. Suarez—a Miami, FL based American urologist/surgeon painlessly blitzed the cancer with high intensity focused ultrasound. Three hours later in the recovery room he informed me that cancer had not metastasized and that I was cancer free.

Widely practiced for years in Europe, Asia, Canada and elsewhere, in the US HIFU, at long last, is in FDA's third stage trials. Hopefully, this important technological advance will soon be available here.

Ira Gollobin
(212) 677-8694
530 F Grand Street
New York, NY 10002

January, 2005

Dear Dr. Bard:

I was diagnosed with prostate cancer in December of 2001 with a Gleason grade of (3+3). The urologist I saw, of course, immediately had me scheduled for surgery in January of 2002. In fact, he told me to go home and think about all that I had been told, and the next thing I knew his office was calling to tell me that I was scheduled for surgery. I told them to cancel that, and I would let them know if I wanted to reschedule. I never did!

I had previously picked up Larry Clapp's book Prostate Health in 90-days-without Drugs or Surgery, and I followed some of Larry's program but not on a regular basis. After the diagnoses I got serious about the program. I did the Ultimate Fast, got on the Budwig diet, changed my diet to include healthy foods and began to have amalgam removed from my mouth. In addition to improvements to my prostate, I feel better and lost approximately 35–40 pounds.

I made my first visit to Dr. Bard in March of 2002 after discussing my situation with Larry Clapp. Dr. Bard examined me and used the Power Doppler sonogram. Everything looked well with no sign of an active tumor. Since this initial visit, I have been seeing Dr. Bard on a regular basis with good reports of each of my visits.

When my PSA results were rising ultimately leading to the prostate cancer diagnosis, I prayed to God for guidance on what course of action to follow. I believe God led me to Larry Clapp and Dr. Bard. I thank God for my continued good health, and I am grateful to Larry and Dr. Bard for their assistance and advice over the past few years.

Rick T.

August 15, 2006

Good morning Dr. Bard,

Since July 17, 2006, I have been taking ProMultiCell 2 capsules 3x per day as you recommended for my prostate cancer. I have type 2 diabetes; I take 1000 mg. of Metformin twice daily, along with 5 mg. of Glipizide once daily. My blood sugar level has been hovering around 130–160, which is higher than I would like. Since I've been taking your ProMultiCell formula, I've noticed a substantial decrease in my blood sugar level. The low was 63 with a high of 125. This morning after fasting it was 103. I've had readings in the morning of 73 and the afternoon and evening of 125–135. Those are great readings. I have not had such low readings for about three years. Last week in the afternoon I checked my blood sugar level it was 165. I took two ProMultiCell capsules and waited for one hour. I took another reading, it was down to 114.

Have you had an experience like this with any other diabetic patients? This is remarkable; I want to thank you for recommending ProMultiCell.

I had HIFU on July 23, 2006; it was performed in Toronto by Dr. George Suarez. It went very well, painless and so far no visible side effects. I have an appointment scheduled with you in January 2007; I am looking forward to seeing you then.

Thank you very much for all your help. Dr. Suarez was right when he said to me that you are a doctor ahead of your time.

Yours truly,

Alan

June 11, 2007

rbard@cancerscan.com

Hola amigas from sunny Canada,

I am doing fine following my HIFU (HIGH INTENSITY FOCUSED ULTRA-SOUND—WWW.USHIFU.COM) procedure to thermally ablate my prostate...along with the bad cells inside of it.

As you can see from the photos, the boys once again did it in style. We enjoyed Niagara Falls on Saturday; then dressed up in our stylish robes (complete with bow ties, dark glasses and dress shirts) to arrive for the surgery. Upon our arrival at the clinic, we informed the receptionist that she would have to select one of the three robed gentlemen for the procedure. Unfortunately for me, my name was on my robe and I was the only candidate wearing the thigh-high (quite fashionable) white stockings.

After a quick photo shoot with the doctors; it was off for the 3 hour procedure. I was awake, but felt intoxicated during the process. No pain during and only slight discomfort after the process. I actually walked across the street to my hotel 2 hours later. Much to my surprise, the nurse to me to eat a nice big meal of what ever I wanted...awesome!

Felt great at night and slept well. The first day after is also going better than expected with minor limitations.

Thanks to dr. Suarez, dr. Barkin and the us and canadian hifu team, this revolutionary process (not yet available in the u.s.) has spared me much pain and has minimized the side effects as compared to conventional prostate surgery.

Pass the word to your male friends that are over the age of 40. It is critical to monitor prostate health, just as a woman would have a breast exam.

Adios for now. I will keep you posted on our travels.

Steve

July 2, 2007

Gentlemen,

My HIFU procedure was done just 3 weeks ago.

Three days after the procedure, I was walking several miles per day.

Six days after the HIFU, I was in Niagara Falls on a helicopter ride and bouncing down the class 5 rapids on the jet boat tour. My girlfriend and I then took a 2 week driving vacation through Montreal and Quebec. There was almost zero post surgical pain, and my lifestyle was barely compromised in the following weeks. The catheter was removed last Friday, and I am urinating as usual. My sexual function returned 10 days following the procedure.

I met with 2 of my friends that had the conventional surgeries 2 years ago. Both are still experiencing post surgical problems. To this point, I am very happy with my choice of the HIFU procedure. Feel free to have any patients call me if they would like to speak with someone that has undergone the HIFU process. I know that it would have settled my nerves prior to surgery to have had the opportunity to speak with someone who had recently experienced the HIFU.

I hope that we can all get together to celebrate a job well done. Again, you are all invited to come down to the Mexico mansion in Acapulco for a relaxing getaway.

Please keep in touch.

Steve Curtis

Text of Major Medical
Prostate Presentation

MRI, MR Spectroscopy and Computed Tomography of Prostate Cancer:
An Update at the 2005 NY Roentgen Society Meeting
Hedvig Hricak, MD, PhD
Chairman, Department of Radiology,
Carroll and Milton Petrie Chair
Memorial Sloan-Kettering Cancer Center
Professor of Radiology,
Weill Medical College of Cornell University

Prostate cancer is the most common cancer and the second leading cause of cancer death in American men. Given its biological heterogeneity, the high prevalence of indolent disease, and the desire for patient-specific treatment design, non-invasive evaluation of tumor prognostic variables, including tumor location, volume, aggressiveness, and extent, continues to be of great clinical interest. Magnetic resonance imaging (MRI) and spectroscopic imaging (MRSI) have demonstrated potential in localizing prostate cancer lesions and assessing tumor aggressiveness and extent. CT has been found helpful in the evaluation of metastatic prostate cancer in radiotherapy planning and treatment follow-up. These modalities can therefore play an important role in risk-adjusted, patient-specific treatment selection, planning and follow-up.

Role of MRI/MRSI in Pretreatment Assessment of Prostate Cancer

Although biopsy is considered the preferred method for prostate cancer detection and characterization, data suggest that even with a threshold PSA value of 4.1 ng per milliliter, biopsy will miss 82% of cancers in men less than 60 years old and 65% of cancers in men over 60. In fact, when biopsy results were compared with radical prostatectomy for sextant tumor localization, the positive predictive value of biopsy was 83.3%, and the negative predictive value was 36.4%. MRI/MRSI is not recommended as a first approach to diagnose prostate cancer but may be useful for directing targeted biopsy, especially for patients with PSA levels indicative of cancer but with negative previous biopsy results; this situation occurs most often with lesions in the anterior peripheral or transition zones (i.e., regions not palpable by digital rectal examination (DRE) and often not routinely sampled during biopsy). The combined use of MRI and MRSI has shown excellent sensitivity and specificity for detecting cancer in the peripheral zone. In a recent study comparing DRE, transrectal ultrasound (TRUS)-guided biopsy and endorectal MRI in the detection and localization of prostate cancer, MRI performed significantly better than DRE in detecting cancer in the apex, mid-gland, and base, and significantly better than TRUS-guided biopsy in the mid gland and base. Unlike either DRE or TRUS-guided biopsy, MRI was also capable of detecting tumor in the transition zone. The use of MRI/MRSI may reduce the rate of false-negative biopsies and hence decrease the need for more extensive biopsy protocols and multiple repeat biopsy procedures.

One of the most challenging characteristics of prostate cancer is its variability in biological aggressiveness. Gleason grade is a good predictor of prostate cancer aggressiveness. However, biopsy prediction of final pathological grade is not reliable. As compared with the histology results from radical prostatectomy, biopsy determined the correct Gleason grade at best in only 58% of cases. MR spectroscopy has the potential to provide a noninvasive means of improving the assessment of prostate cancer aggressiveness. It has been shown that the ratio of choline+creatine to citrate in a prostate cancer lesion correlates with the Gleason grade, with the elevation of choline and reduction of citrate indicating increased tumor aggressiveness.

MRI/MRSI has also been shown to aid in determining the local extent of prostate cancer. A study by Wang et al. has shown that MRI contributes significant incremental value to clinical variables in the prediction of extracapsular extension. On MRI, the criteria for extracapsular extension include a contour deformity with a step-off or angulated margin; an irregular bulge or edge retraction; a breech of the capsule with evidence of direct tumor extension; obliteration of the recto-prostatic angle; and asymmetry of the neurovascular bundles. While transaxial planes of section are essential in the evaluation of extracapsular invasion, the combination of transaxial and coronal plane images facilitates the diagnosis of extracapsular extension. The addition of volumetric data from MRSI to the anatomic display of MRI significantly improves the evaluation of extracapsular cancer extension and decreases interobserver variability.

MRI is also useful for demonstrating seminal vesicle invasion. The criteria for seminal vesicle invasion on MRI include contiguous low signal-intensity tumor extension from the base of the gland into the seminal vesicles; tumor extension along the ejaculatory duct (non-visualization of the ejaculatory duct); asymmetric decrease in the signal intensity of the seminal vesicles; and decreased conspicuity of the seminal vesicle wall on T2-weighted images. Combined axial, coronal and sagittal planes of section facilitate evaluation of seminal vesical and bladder neck invasion.

Over the past four years, studies on the use MRI in the evaluation of prostate cancer have obtained more promising results than did initial studies. The diagnostic performance for experienced readers has improved, with reported accuracy reaching between 75% and 93%. The recently reported sensitivities of MRI for detection of extracapsular extension and seminal vesicle invasion and the high specificity of MRI in excluding extracapsular tumors far exceed the values reported for both TRUS and CT. However, it has been shown that the incremental value of MRI in predicting extracapsular extension is significant only when interpretation is performed by a radiologist with substantial experience in MRI and thorough clinical knowledge of the disease. This suggests that the recent improvement in the performance of MRI is likely due to increased reader experience in addition to the maturation of MRI technology (e.g. faster imaging sequences, more powerful gradient coils, and post-processing image correction) and better understanding of morphologic criteria used to diagnose extracapsular extension or seminal vesicle invasion.

Computed Tomography

The main role of CT in prostate cancer management is in the assessment of metastatic disease in the lymph nodes, visceral organs and bones. Due to the lack of soft-tissue contrast, CT has limited value in initial tumor staging, unless advanced disease is suspected. However, it is useful in radiotherapy treatment planning in patients with locally advanced prostate cancer and also in treatment follow-up. The majority of patients with newly diagnosed prostate cancer are at low risk for metastases, hence the diagnostic yield of CT is relatively low in these patients. CT is not recommended for patients with a PSA < 20 ng/ml, a Gleason score < 7, or a clinical stage < T3 as the likelihood of lymph node metastasis and systemic disease is very low. At present, according to the American Urology Association guidelines, there is no indication for CT in a patient with a PSA level < 25 ng/ml.

CT Imaging Findings in Local Tumor Staging

Although there is no recent literature on the CT appearance of organ-confined prostate cancer, in our personal experience with multi-slice CT, prostate cancer appears as an area of low attenuation compared to the surrounding normal prostate tissue. CT can be useful as a baseline examination prior to radiation or medical therapy in clinically high-risk patients with grossly advanced local disease demonstrated by established extracapsular disease, gross seminal vesicle invasion, or invasion of surrounding structures including bladder, rectum, levator ani muscles, or pelvic floor. Such patients will also be at risk for lymph node metastases, which may be assessed concurrently.

Detection of Metastatic Disease on CT

Currently, the diagnosis of nodal metastases on CT is made based on nodal size. However, the correlation between nodal enlargement and metastatic involvement is poor. Using a short axis diameter of 1.0 cm as a cut off has resulted in sensitivity values between 25% and 85% and specificity between 66% and 100%. Oyen et al reported a significant improvement in both sensitivity and specificity (78% and 100% respectively) with lowering of the size threshold to 0.7 cm and performance of fine needle aspiration (FNA) of the suspicious nodes. However, neither decreased size criteria, nor the use of FNA has been widely accepted. Neither CT nor MRI can be used to rule out lymph node metastases, especially in normal-sized lymph nodes. However, recently, high-resolution MRI with lymphotropic superparamagnetic nanoparticles has demonstrated promising results in diagnosis of metastasis within normal-sized lymph nodes.

Knowledge of the anatomical nodal spread is essential for proper image interpretation. The regional nodes for prostate cancer that are designated as N1 in the TNM classification are pelvic nodes, including obturator, iliac (internal and external), and sacral (lateral, presacral, promontory) nodes. Metastatic lymph nodes (M1) are common iliac, paraaortic, mesenteric and mediastinal nodes. Prior to any form of therapy, nodal disease usually progresses in step-wise fashion, such that retroperitoneal, mesenteric or mediastinal nodal disease is very unusual in the absence of pelvic lymphadenopathy and more likely to be due to coexistent malignancy (e.g., lymphoma). However, in patients with disease recurrence following radical prostatectomy the usual pattern of vertical node spread is not maintained in almost 75% of the patients. The majority of these patients would have had previous lymph node dissection at the time of radical prostatectomy and thus only retroperitoneal lymphadenopathy would be detected at CT.

CT is also valuable in the evaluation of visceral and bone metastasis. Bone metastases from prostate cancer are usually sclerotic due to osteoblastic reaction, but a mixed lytic-sclerotic pattern can occasionally be observed. However, bone scintigraphy and MRI are superior to CT in since metastasis after chemo/radiation treatment can appear larger, thus leading to incorrect estimation of disease progression.

Abstract

Abstract of Dean Ornish, MD 2005 paper in the Journal of Urology

Title: Intensive Lifestyle Changes May Affect the Progression of Prostate Cancer

Conclusions:

"Patients…maintain comprehensive lifestyle changes…resulting in significant decreases in serum PSA"

"…substantially decreased growth of LNCaP prostate cancer cells was seen when such cells were incubated in the presence of serum from those who made lifestyle changes. These findings suggest that intensive changes in diet and lifestyle may beneficially affect the progression of early prostate cancer."

Internet Nutritional Resources:

Arbor Clinical Nutrition Updates
http://www.nutritionupdates.org/

Center for Responsible Nutrition
http://www.crnusa.org/

American Holistic Medical Association
www.holisticmedicine.org

Consumer Lab:
http://consumerlab.com

FDA Center for Food Safety & Applied Nutrition
http://www.cfsan.fda.gov/

Food and Nutrition Information Center
http://www.nal.usda.gov/fnic

NIH National Center for Complementary and Alternative Medicine:
http://nccam.nih.gov

NIH Office of Dietary Supplements
http://dietary-suplements.info.nih.gov

Breaking news on supplements and nutrition
http://www.nutraingredients-usa.com/

SupplementWatch
http://www.supplementwatch.com/

The American Herbal Pharmacopoeia
http://www.herbal-ahp.org/

Harvard Women's healthwatch
http://www.health.harvard.edu/newsletters/Harvard_Womens_Health_Watch.htm

Mayo Clinic Newsletter
www.mayoclinic.com

Publications

Journals and Magazines

Alternative and Complementary Therapies
Mary Ann Liebert, Inc. Publishers
2 Madison Ave,
Larchmont, NY 10538
(914) 834-3100
www.liebertpub.com
info@liebertpub.com

Journal of Medicinal Foods
www.liebertonline.com/jmf

Alternative Therapies in Health and Medicine
InnoVision Communications, LLC
2995 Wilderness Place, Suite 205
Boulder, CO 80301
(303) 440-7402
www.alternative-therapies.com

EXPLORE
The Journal of Science and Healing
Elsevier Inc.
360 Park Avenue South
New York, NY 10010
Tel: (800) 654-2452
www.explorejournal.com/

HerbalGram
American Botanical Council
PO BOX 2016600
Austin, TX 78720
(512) 926-4900
www.herbalgram.org

Newsletters and Other Periodicals

Center for Medical Consumer
239 Thompson St.
New York, NY 10012
www.medicalconsumers.org
medconsumers@earthlink.net

The Collaborative on Health and the Environment
c/o Commonweal
PO Box 316, Bolinas, CA 94924
www.healthandenvironment.org

Environmental Nutrition
P.O. Box 420234
Palm Coast, FL 32142-0234
800-829-5384
www.environmentalnutrition.com/

Other Resources

American Botanical Council
PO Box 201660
Austin, TX 78720-1660
(512) 331-886 (800)-373-7105
www.herbalgram.org

FREE BONUS POWERPOINT

From
The Biofoundation for Angiogenesis Research and Development

Non-invasive Cancer Treatments

See Why:

PSA Blood Test is 2% Accurate

Random Biopsies Miss 80% of Cancer

3-D Doppler Ultrasound finds 95% of
Clinically Significant Tumors

MRI Screening can Avert Biopsies

Image Guided Treatments are Safer

Download Powerpoint at
http://www.cancerscan.com